UNDERSTAND DIGITAL WELLNESS IN THE OVERWHELMING DIGITAL AGE

LEARN HOW TO IMPROVE DIGITAL HABITS

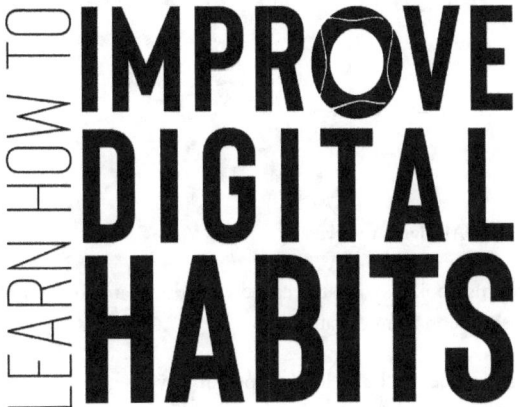

IN ORDER TO NAVIGATE THE MANY MENTAL HEALTH CHALLENGES CAUSED BY TECH

JESSIE FIELDS

© Copyright 2022 - All rights reserved.

The contents of this book may not be reproduced, duplicated or transmitted without direct written permission from the author.

Under no circumstances will any legal responsibility or blame be held against the publisher for any reparation, damages, or monetary loss due to the information herein, either directly or indirectly.

Legal Notice:

This book is copyright protected. This is only for personal use. You cannot amend, distribute, sell, use, quote or paraphrase any part or the content within this book without the consent of the author.

Disclaimer Notice:

Please note the information contained within this document is for educational and entertainment purposes only. Every attempt has been made to provide accurate, up to date, and reliable complete information. No warranties of any kind are expressed or implied. Readers acknowledge that the author is not engaging in the rendering of legal, financial, medical or professional advice. The content of this book has been derived from various sources. Please consult a licensed professional before attempting any techniques outlined in this book.

By reading this document, the reader agrees that under no circumstances is the author responsible for any losses, direct or indirect, which are incurred as a result of the use of information contained within this document, including, but not limited to, —errors, omissions, or inaccuracies.

Contents

Introduction	1
1. What Is Digital Wellness?	11
2. The Age of Overwhelm	23
3. The Myth of Multitasking	33
4. Digital Distractions	45
5. Everything's Fighting for Your Attention	55
6. Digital Clutter and Digital Hoarding	67
7. Dealing with Mental Load	77
8. Coping with Isolation	87
Conclusion	103

Introduction

Digital Detox has become a big business in recent years. Not only has it become an increasingly common Web search topic, but there has also been a sharp rise in books, newspaper articles, and web pages devoted to how people can get as far away from digital devices as they possibly could. At least for a little while.

This information led David Kushner to found Camp No Counselors, a weekend camp for people twenty years and over where phones are not welcome. Inspired by a weekend trip Kushner took with friends in 2013, Camp No Counselors is meant to resurrect the memory of summer camp. Though they unintentionally picked a site with no cell service for that first outing, they quickly discovered that "getting away from it all" made their camp experience even more enjoyable.

As a result, the Camp No Counselors group, founded by Kushner, now makes it a firm rule that cell phones need to be left behind in the bunks. Meanwhile, everyone participates in activities such as archery, dodgeball, and arts and crafts. "People often say it's the best part of the weekend because you're allowed to get yourself off that leash," Kushner said in a recent interview. "Sometimes, you feel phantom signals from your pocket for the first day or so.

But it's so nice to be able to escape again. It's a luxury in this time to be able to escape a lot of the pressures of the real world. People love to drop that for just a weekend."

Though the COVID-19 pandemic has put a crimp in Kushner's business (along with the rest of the travel industry), the demand for digital detox camps has not subsided. As a result, places that once had trouble attracting tourists due to the lack of cell service and Wi-Fi are now advertising these features to cash in on the digital detox tourism industry.

For the past two decades, the entire world has been part of a bold new experiment never seen before in history. Along with the rise of an increasingly accessible Internet, smartphones have become virtually universal with people of all ages, while other digital devices, including tablets, iPods, and smartwatches, are competing for our attention as well.

According to the 2018 Internet Trends survey (Meeker, 2018), the average adult American spends 5.9 hours a day engaged in some form of digital media. Of that, 3.3 hours are taken up by smartphones or other mobile devices (checking for messages, using the Internet, texting, email, or phone calls), 2.1 hours are spent on desktop or laptop computers, and the rest on other digital devices.

Even parts of the world that have traditionally lagged industrialized nations in communications technology have now leapfrogged into the future, with cell phone towers being found in the most unlikely places powered by solar panels. An estimated 3.8 billion people are smartphone users, and 4.66 billion are internet users as well.

This digital revolution has already transformed our lives, with entire industries springing up, including digital streaming services and social media providers, such as Netflix, Facebook, and others, and companies like Uber and Airbnb transforming the transportation and travel industry. And the revolution is only just beginning.

But where is this brave new world taking us? There is already an entire generation of children, adolescents, and young adults who have never known a world without digital devices, and, even for the rest of us, the memory of a pre-Internet world is fading rapidly. Unfortunately, however, the same technological changes that are making life so much easier in many ways are also creating new challenges and risks to our mental and physical health, resulting from the "digital overwhelm" that few people are fully prepared to handle.

In this book we will examine many mental health challenges arising from digital technology and what they will mean for you and your children. Along with introducing you to the concept of digital wellness, you will also learn more about the iGen generation and why young people seem much less happy than ever before.

We will further explore "Facebook depression" and cyberbullying, as well as the new epidemic of hate speech, mean-spirited comments, unwanted contacts, and misunderstandings fuelled by the anonymity provided by the Internet, which seems to be eroding mental health for people of all ages.

We will also look at how the recent pandemic is transforming how we work and play by making us more dependent on the Internet and digital devices to stay in touch with friends and family. Why does this seem to be eroding the social networks we depend on to keep us emotionally healthy? And why is remote working, once declared to be the perfect solution for working parents and people wanting to avoid long commutes, not as beneficial as many hoped initially?

In later chapters, we will also explore the meaning of "technostress" and why we are in the "age of overwhelm". We will also examine related concepts such as "techno-anxiety" and "digital burnout" and why these are becoming increasingly real problems for large segments of society. That means learning more about the nature of stress and the three stages of the stress adaptation process so that we can avoid the long-term health problems too much technostress can bring.

Then we will look at the myth of multitasking and why trying to do too many things at once will only slow us down and lead to mistakes. That includes the dangers of distracted driving and why motor vehicle accidents caused by texting and other digital distractions are becoming more common. However, that is only one example of how digital distractions can undermine our ability to function at work, school, and home.

We will also explore what cognitive psychology says about how memory works and why "the Magic Number Seven Plus or Minus Two:" helps explain why our brains don't work like computers. We will also get into why digital devices are screwing up our sleep schedules and why children are losing so much valuable sleep time because of digital devices in their bedrooms.

Next, what is FOMO, also known as the fear of missing out? While everybody likes to stay informed, why is the rise of the Internet and social media imposing far more challenges than ever before? Are other people's fun and positive news stories making your own life seem less interesting as a result? Why are survey studies showing that people with a greater fear of missing out are experiencing mental and physical health problems?

For that matter, why are more parents than ever worrying about the amount of digital screen time their children are getting and how this is affecting them? And why are so many of these parents admitting to experiencing significant problems with digital distraction themselves? What are the teachers saying about digital devices in the classrooms and how this interferes with their ability to teach students? And why are they reporting that the number of children with psychological, social, and behavioral issues has risen sharply over the past five years?

Next, we will explore the "attention economy" and why competing for your attention has become a multi-billion-dollar industry in recent years. Shutting them out is so much harder to do these days with all the pop-up ads, specialized ringtones, and text messages demanding your time and attention at any moment of the day or night. A handful of multinational companies such as Facebook, Alphabet (better known as Google), and several Chinese corporations dominate the attention economy (at least for now). There are also billions of websites and countless spammers targeting us whenever we turn on a digital device, all trying to pull us in and grab our attention.

What about smartphone and social media addiction? Is it possible that we can become addicted to our digital devices in the same way that people can become addicted to gambling, overeating, or shopping? Based on the available research completed to date, the answer appears to be "yes." Though there is still some controversy, mainly since researchers are divided on how to define social media or internet addiction, young people appear particularly vulnerable because they were introduced to social media and the Internet at a much younger age and are more comfortable with communicating that way.

It isn't just social media and the Internet that can lead to people becoming dependent. There is also the smartphone which has already become the most popular digital device. Later in this book, you will learn about the "Digital Dozen" and how digital addiction makes us more isolated than ever.

We will also look at "digital clutter" and the dangers of "e-hoarding." How clogged is your email Inbox, and how many pictures, music files, videos, text files, or plain junk is currently on your computer, most of which you are unlikely ever to look at again? Especially in an era of cloud computing and multi-terabyte hard drivers, the average computer user can accumulate tens of thousands of files that are never deleted because they "might become useful someday." For that matter, the average inbox contains 102 unread, and 331 read emails, most of them long since obsolete but which people are still reluctant to delete for whatever reason. Even if we dismiss the importance of this kind of digital clutter, what are the long-term environmental costs considering the electricity needs of storage systems worldwide? And will the problem grow even worse in the future? That means learning to embrace digital minimalism and making it a regular part of your routine.

We will also look at the complex problem of mental load and why being preoccupied with other issues can seriously undermine our ability to function at work and in school. How much of a psychological toll can occur due to being unable to 'switch off' or relax, considering all the digital reminders we get of work still needing to be done? And what about decision fatigue resulting from the thousands of decisions that the average person makes every day? Why are we better able to make crucial decisions in the morning rather than late in the afternoon? For that matter, why are health professionals and air flight control operators, among others, starting to take decision fatigue more seriously as a way of avoiding accidents and employee burnout? How do digital devices such as computers, smartphones, and tablets affect this growing problem with mental load? Will the massive influx of new time-saving and labor-saving apps aimed at making life easier, both at work and at home make our lives easier? We will cover this later in the book.

Are digital devices making us more isolated, especially since the pandemic? And what are hikikomori, and what might this growing social problem in Japan and other Asian countries mean for our own future? The final chapter takes a sobering look at the increasing trend of isolation linked to digital devices, especially in young people, as actual face-to-face social contact becomes less important due to social media, email, texting, TikTok videos, etc. Is it because of digital addiction? Or are younger generations generally becoming lonelier due to too much social media use?

We will look at research showing that adolescents currently spend far less time on face-to-face interactions with people their own age than twenty years ago. This means spending less time hanging out, going to parties, dating, going to movies, etc. As you might expect, many of these same adolescents report a sharp rise in reported loneliness from 2011 onward, especially for those reporting high social media use.

Even for adults, research suggests a strong link between social media use and loneliness. And this works both ways. Not only are lonely people more likely to turn to social media as a way of forming social connections, but the time spent on social media can also increase loneliness.

Yes, it is undoubtedly possible to join different online communities and to interact with hundreds, if not thousands, of like-minded people across the world. But unfortunately, there is still a trade-off between the many relationships that can be formed online and the actual *quality* of those relationships. Also, consider the kind of online abuse to which even children and adolescents can be exposed.

This sort of online harassment is prevalent for women and members of sexual or racial minority groups, given that many harassers take advantage of being anonymous to engage in crudely extremist language and threats. This includes cyberbullying behavior such as posting rumors, making crude sexual remarks, hate speech, or releasing personal information, as well as revealing images aimed at humiliating victims.

Considering that at least half of all young people have experienced cyberbullying in some form, it is still the ones who spend the most time online who are particularly vulnerable. As a result, victims of cyberbullying often develop a lower sense of self-esteem. They can also become depressed and suicidal if they are unable to fight back against anonymous harassment. This can make them become even more isolated and avoid family and friends who might help them cope. Though an estimated twenty to forty percent of adolescents are believed to be victims of cyberbullying worldwide, the actual number will likely never be known since many victims hide their abuse.

Along with documenting the dark side of digital technology, we will also be looking at ways that you and your children can learn to get this digital overwhelm under control. Along with making digital detox a regular part of your life, whether, through weekend getaways at places like Camp No Counselor or something you can do on your own, you will also learn how to deal with digital clutter, digital distractions, and technostress. We will also discuss how to set basic ground rules for yourself about where and when to use your digital devices and how to insulate yourself from annoying pop-up notifications, ringtones, and spam mail. That means knowing when to turn those devices *off* if you need time to relax or get a little more sleep.

We will also look at how to ask for help when dealing with online harassment, including cyberbullying and hate speech, as well as what to do if your digital addiction is stronger than you initially realized. There are resources out there, but you need to know where to look for them, whether online or in your community.

Remember, we are still in the early stages of this digital revolution, and you may not be prepared for what is coming next. New changes, such as the Internet of Things and quantum computing, will keep on transforming life as we know it, and it is vital to prepare yourself now as much as you can. Whether you like it or not, you and your children will be living in a digital world for the rest of your lives. How you learn to handle it is up to you.

Chapter One

What Is Digital Wellness?

In 2012 University of San Diego psychologist Jean Twenge first observed a disturbing new trend in her research. A well-known authority in research looking at happiness and psychological well-being (i.e., emotional health and overall life satisfaction) across different generations, Dr. Twenge had previously published numerous studies looking at self-esteem and happiness in young people, including children, adolescents, and young adults. Her research findings, along with those of many other researchers in her field, had shown a steady rise in psychological well-being among young people over the previous four decades. During 1991-2012, reported levels of psychological well-being in adolescents either remained the same or rose steadily.

But then she began noticing an abrupt change in how teens described their behavior and emotional states. Starting in 2012 and continuing through to 2016, survey results for young people showed a dramatic drop in most aspects of psychological well-being. Along with overall life satisfaction, the results also showed reductions in how satisfied they were with their friendships, how happy they were with the government, their personal safety, the level of fun they experienced, and how satisfied they were with their family relationships. Personal happiness and self-esteem also declined significantly.

This new trend meant that the rise in well-being and life satisfaction Dr. Twenge had seen in young people over previous decades had rapidly evaporated. While young people seemed to be growing steadily happier over time, they were now much more vulnerable to depression and social anxiety issues. As she would later note in a 2017 article in The Atlantic, "In all my analyses of generational data—some reaching back to the 1930s—I had never seen anything like it."

Introducing the iGen Generation

Despite initially believing that this change was a statistical anomaly, Dr. Twenge quickly ruled this explanation out. Instead, for reasons that she and her fellow researchers were only beginning to understand, something occurred around 2012 that had far more impact than any significant social change reported over the past eight decades. That included generations affected by wars, social upheavals, economic booms and busts, and political unrest; none of them had impacted young people as severely as what was happening over the past eight years.

Dr. Twenge began interviewing young people to learn how their lives had changed to explore this strange new trend. One common denominator quickly emerged: the rise of the smartphone and social media. As part of what she termed the "IGen generation," all children born since 1995 grew up in a world in which smartphones and other digital devices were universally available.

While previous generations, including Millennials, were also affected by the digital transformation of modern society, they could at least remember what the world was like before digital devices came on the scene. But the oldest members of the iGen generation were still pre-teens when the first iPhone arrived in 2007 and only a little older when the first iPads came out in 2010.

Perhaps as importantly, the parents of these children seemed largely oblivious to what was happening. As a result, aside from some initial controversy over "screen time," parents ensured that their children had the best and most expensive digital gadgets to prevent them from becoming "digital have-nots."

Since there may be other culprits at work, digital devices alone may not deserve the complete blame. Still, the iGen generation faces challenges their parents or grandparents never encountered when they were growing up. Not only had there been a general drop in face-to-face social interactions among adolescents in recent years, but they also seemed to be getting less sleep due to the presence of smartphones and other digital devices in their bedrooms. In addition, the need to stay in touch with the outside world, play video games, or catch up on social media often meant long hours spent on smartphones and computers, all of which cut into the number of hours they might otherwise spend sleeping.

Understand Facebook Depression & Cyberbullying

There is also the issue of "Facebook depression," a term originating from a 2011 report released by the American Academy of Pediatrics (Schurgin et al., 2011). The term was introduced to describe the emotional impact social media, gaming, video, and blogging sites can have on young people. For example, sites such as Facebook, Instagram, and Twitter allow users to post status updates, wall posts, photos, and videos that can make other young users feel unpopular, whether intentionally or unintentionally.

These sites also allow for anonymous postings, which make them prime breeding grounds for cyberbullying, especially when users post pictures, videos, or other content deliberately intended to humiliate or defame others, whether the cyberbully knows the victim or not. Indeed, we have seen a proliferation of racist, sexists, homophobic, or other forms of derogatory comments that could be legally branded as harassment if the poster could be identified. As such, the result is often devastating, especially for young people who already have issues with low self-esteem or social anxiety, which can lead to depression and even suicide in many cases.

One graphic example occurred in 2013 when 17-year-old Rehtaeh Parsons hanged herself after online photographs emerged showing an alleged gang rape that occurred a year earlier. Once the rape became public knowledge in her small town, Rehtaeh was deemed to be at fault, and she was bombarded with text and Facebook messages pressuring her for sex. She hanged herself soon afterward and, though paramedics saved her life, was left brain-dead and only died when her parents decided to take her off life support. Though her case generated considerable publicity and new cyberbullying legislation in her native Nova Scotia, few other jurisdictions have followed suit.

Though it is still hard to prove an actual link between online activities and emotional problems in young people, recent research shows that 82 percent of young people studied have had numerous negative experiences on Facebook. These findings include episodes of bullying, mean-spirited comments, unwanted contacts, and misunderstandings resulting from Facebook posts. Not surprisingly, users reporting negative Facebook experiences were more than three times as likely to develop depression than those who did not report such incidents (Rosenthal et al., 2016). As lead researcher Samantha Rosenthal pointed out, "I think it's important that people take interactions on social media seriously and don't think of it as somehow less impactful because it's a virtual experience as opposed to an in-person experience," she said. "It's a different forum that has real emotional consequences."

Facebook has implemented safeguards intended to prevent abuse, including the ability to "unfriend" or block harassers. However, as this is difficult to police, many victims can be forced to abandon social media altogether. Especially considering how easy it is for harassers to set up bogus accounts to continue their harassment. Still, this is hardly an option for a generation increasingly dependent on social media and the Internet. If anything, they have few real alternatives but to "grin and bear it" as much as possible and report people who are too blatant in their harassment.

For young adults, there are also risks that can arise from the use of dating and "hookup" apps such as Tinder, Grinder, Match, and OkCupid. While most users agree about the potential dangers involved, more young people than ever are turning to these online sites to find dates. In a later chapter, we will explore the risks involved, including posting personal information about themselves, which they might never share under other circumstances.

Boomers, Millennials, and the Digital Revolution

It isn't just the iGen generation that is being affected by the proliferation of digital devices. According to a 2017 Stress in America survey, nearly all adults (99 percent) own at least one electronic device (including a television). In addition, almost nine in 10 (86 percent) own a computer, 74 percent own an internet-connected smartphone, and 55 percent own a tablet. Furthermore, 86 percent of the more than 3000 American adults participating in the study reported constantly checking their social media accounts, email, and texts each day. (APA, 2017).

That same study makes an intriguing distinction between the "constant checkers" and the "non-constant checkers" regarding overall stress. You won't find it surprising that constant checkers are much more likely than non-constant checkers to view technology as a significant source of stress, with a minority describing it as potentially harmful. That includes the emotional upset they experience from political and cultural discussions and the stress resulting from technical problems that disrupt their digital contact.

Many of the same issues affecting younger users apply to adults as well, especially when dealing with mean-spirited, harassing, or otherwise upsetting content. Unfortunately, for women and sexual minorities, cyber-harassment and cyber-stalking are all too familiar, and complaints to the social media sites themselves rarely change anything.

The recent pandemic has added to this digital trend due to a sharp rise in remote working with countless employees carrying out team assignments, participating in digital meetings, and working independently with minimal physical contact with employers and fellow employees. Remote working thus means more screen time than ever and increasing dependence on smartphones and computers. Not only does this play havoc with a proper work-life balance, but there is no actual "off" switch allowing employees to separate themselves from their work responsibilities.

As a result, it is hardly surprising that many employees report spending half their waking hours glued to their screens and checking their email at all hours of the day. This means even those of us who are not "iGens" encounter the same problems with loss of sleep, increased anxiety, loss of social contact with colleagues, and a rise in digital scrutiny with supposedly private posts being used as grounds for job termination or demotion.

All of this has a significant effect on worker self-esteem and well-being in general, so, understandably, a July 2020 survey by Monster.com reported that two-thirds of remote employees described burnout symptoms. Since this represents a 20 percent rise from just a few months earlier, you can imagine how this developed throughout the pandemic. The entire concept of a "nine to five" work schedule seems obsolete mainly, with more workers than ever-adapting their work schedules to accommodate other responsibilities such as child-care. But even this supposed flexibility is becoming a myth as employers increasingly expect their remote workers to be "on-call" at all hours of the day (or night).

A 2020 study by the National Bureau of Economic Research surveying 3.1 million workers worldwide showed that the average workday is 48.5 minutes longer for workers at home compared to just a year earlier. Also, the number of meetings attended by remote workers has risen about 13%, and people sent an average of 1.4 more emails per day to their colleagues (DeFillipis et al., 2020). While the study focused primarily on the impact of the pandemic on remote workers, there are few tangible signs that the changes brought on by pandemic lockdowns will ever return to pre-pandemic levels. Like it or not, this is the new normal for remote workers, and it probably will not be changing back for the foreseeable future.

Distracted Driving and the New Digital Reality

Suppose you doubt that we are becoming more dependent on our smartphones and other digital devices. In that case, data from the National Highway Traffic Safety Administration shows that an estimated 78 percent of all crashes and 65 percent of near-crashes in the United States alone were due to distracted driving. Particularly distracted driving involving smartphones. For that matter, more recent studies showed that one out of every six fatal crashes in the United States might be due to distracted driving.

Though most of these accidents appear to involve young people, the use of digital devices while driving has become increasingly common for drivers of all ages. This is especially true when you consider the popularity of global positioning system (GPS) devices for navigation, not to mention the ease of using smartphones to check appointments or call or text friends and family. All these activities involve having drivers shift their attention away from driving, even briefly. Considering that driving is one of the riskiest activities that people engage in daily, even a brief distraction may be enough to cause an accident or near-accident.

Unfortunately, many driving activities can seem virtually automatic for experienced drivers who might feel confident enough to try "multitasking:" by doing other activities simultaneously. Even something as benign as listening to music might cause a driver not to notice in time if traffic conditions have changed.

While automobile companies have tried to reduce the risk of distracted driving by introducing Bluetooth technology in newer model cars, distracted driving is still a risk. This will likely worsen as drivers continue to "push the limit" of what is possible or safe while driving.

What is Digital Wellness

What can we do about the problems caused by digital devices considering that the iGen generation, not to mention the rest of us, will be living in a digital world for the rest of our lives? Indeed, more companies than ever realize that it makes good economic sense to shift away from office-based work and inflexible work hours towards having employees working at home. So, are we inevitably bound for a more impersonal, more dismal cyber-future? Or is there a way that we can learn to live with the digital world?

All of this brings us to the increasingly important concept of *digital wellness*, i.e., the state of our mental and physical health in a digital age. More specifically, what we can do, both as parents and as digital consumers, to ensure that we can prevent the various mental health issues that can stem from the overuse of digital technology. Though researchers and media outlets have been warning about the mental health risks of digital devices for years (Twenge, 2017), many companies are only now acknowledging the mental and physical health issues their remote workers face and providing treatment options to help them cope.

This means teaching employees and everyone else feeling overwhelmed by their digital devices how to take charge of their life online. Scheduling "digital detox" periods regularly can be an important part of the digital wellness process. Though many people, whether iGens or not, may be uncomfortable with cutting themselves from social media and the Internet entirely, there are some gentler alternatives. These can include changing the setting on your smartphone to turn off "push" notifications whenever you get a new email, text, or post. For that matter, you can try rediscovering the benefits of simple conversation during family dinners by banning smartphones from the dining table until after you finish eating. Granted, hearing about what your parents or siblings did with their day may not seem as exciting as the latest YouTube video or hot meme, but it is a lot more emotionally satisfying.

You can also set limits on how much time you spend on social media or the Internet each day. For that matter, you can try limiting the amount of time you spend watching television or playing video games as well. But, unfortunately, far too many parents report feeling increasingly isolated from their children due to the amount of time their children spend online. Moreover, given their own tendency to check email five times a day, they also find themselves unable to curb their own online habits, let alone rein in their children's screen time.

There is also the matter of "digital clutter". Is your Desktop filling up with files you no longer need or cannot even recognize? Is your computer or smartphone filling up with apps or programs that you no longer need and are obsolete? Do you have megabytes of memory devoted to programs, documents, videos, or photos that you haven't looked at in ages and likely never need again? While it might seem tempting to delete as much of this as possible, far too many people seem determined to keep them, hoping that they might need them again someday. In a real sense, people like that have crossed the line into "digital hoarding", which while seemingly harmless, means accumulating years and even decades' worth of obsolete files that take up useless space.

It is also essential that you start educating yourself about the potential dangers of being online. Along with the inevitable spam mail and phishing attempts that everyone experiences, you also need to add new terms to your vocabulary, such as "doxing," "catfishing", and "swatting", to name just a few. It is also essential to maintain effective boundaries regarding the information you share online, especially considering the increased risk of identity theft and the risk of leaving yourself open to cyberstalking and other threats. We will be exploring these different dangers and how to protect yourself later in this book.

In this chapter, I have discussed many of the radical social and cultural changes over the past decades with the rise of digital technologies such as smartphones, tablets, digital streaming services, and social media. Despite the potential of this new technology for fostering greater social interactivity and information sharing, we are also seeing the emotional effects of too much social media and internet contact. Though our world is becoming increasingly digital, with billions already online and billions more likely to follow over the next decade, we need to come to terms with the overwhelming amount of data we are expected to process and what this means in terms of mental health. Young people appear especially vulnerable given how dependent they have become on this new technology and how digital devices have transformed how they interact with friends, family, and total strangers. I also introduced you to the concept of digital wellness and what it can mean in helping people of all ages stay mentally and physically healthy in an increasingly digital age. We will be exploring all the different ways of applying digital wellness techniques in the chapters that follow.

Chapter Two

The Age of Overwhelm

When Silicon Valley psychotherapist Craig Brod wrote his 1984 book, Technostress, he tried to sound an alarm about the very similar symptoms he was seeing in many of his clients. They were all dealing with high technology, be they computer coders or CEOs. "With a typewriter, there were time and motion interruptions when you tore up a piece of paper or hit the carriage return," he said in his book. "Then comes this wonderful technology that alters time. You can work for hours being almost motionless and basically, you are hooked into this machine."

This disappearance of a "human sense of time" alarmed Brod most since he saw it virtually everywhere that humans interacted with machines. Whether it was at an ATM when humans did their banking or at the checkout line as clerks ran groceries over a computer scanner with almost no conversation whatsoever. For that matter, most offices were so computerized that even people who sat next to each other preferred to send emails rather than chat directly. As he concluded sadly, "we are producing this automated society not meeting our needs for personal contact, for a human sense of time. I even have patients who ask me how much time they should spend with their children." In concluding his book, Brod foresaw an eventual revolt if the technostress he was warning about was not dealt with since "we are automating the human element out of our lives."

In the decades since Brod's book was published, the term he coined, "technostress," has become part of our everyday vocabulary. Along with related terms such as "digital overwhelm" and "digital burnout," they are all frequently used to describe the mental health issues that can stem from the growing use of digital technologies and how they have come to dominate our everyday lives. Not only do digital technologies shape how we communicate with others at home and in the workplace (via smartphones, email, texting, etc.), but most workplaces are now dependent on software-based work environments and work processes (including enterprise resource planning software).

We have also seen a radical shift in how most people do their jobs with the rise of the gig economy and the corresponding decline in the "nine-to-five" employment model that dominated work and home life in the last century. And we are on the cusp of an even more significant transformation with the Internet of Things (IoT) that may make us even more dependent on technology than anyone ever dreamed back in the 20th century. But, unfortunately, we are still faced with many of the same problems related to technology overuse that Brod warned about back in 1984.

What is Technostress?

In much the same way that technology has snowballed since Brod's time, the term he introduced has also changed. According to more recent research into the field (Salanova, et al., 2013), technostress is now considered to have different dimensions, including:

- Techno-anxiety – This refers to the fear or emotional agitation that can arise from using a digital device. This includes the fear of making a mistake and accidentally deleting important information or the feeling of uncertainty that can come from using a digital device without the necessary experience.

- Techno-addiction – This is a technological version of workaholism. Techno-addiction stems from being unable to disconnect from work-related use of digital devices, including checking and rechecking emails, text messages, phone messages, etc., even outside of regular business hours. Many techno-addicts are no longer able to maintain a healthy work-life balance and find themselves incapable of turning their work-life "off", even temporarily, because digital devices have invaded their lives so completely. They also experience frequent conflicts with other family members and friends as their fear of missing out on important messages disrupts the home life that might otherwise provide a release from job stress. Techno-addiction can also include the "nomophobia" that people often experience when they can no longer access their digital devices, whether through being out of range of a cell tower or being in a forced "digital detox" due to friends or family members.

- Techno-strain – This refers to the often-cynical attitude that many people have towards the growing use of technology in the workplace. Like the cynicism that often comes with employee burnout, this kind of techno-strain usually occurs when workers are exhausted or discouraged because they see their jobs as being more vulnerable.

- Techno-inadequacy – Mainly due to changing workloads, many workers may find themselves trying to cope with chronic, overwhelming demands on their time. Along with becoming increasingly exhausted by all the demands being placed on them, workers often begin feeling more inadequate when they can no longer do jobs as effectively as they had in the past. In addition, since many of these same workers are also growing older, they may lose confidence in their skills as workers and become generally discouraged due to the fear of losing their jobs because they are no longer able to do the work. Another aspect of techno-inadequacy is techno-complexity, the fear that the technology at work is becoming so complicated that they will no longer be able to understand it.

Because organizations constantly rely on new information, they are continually upgrading the technology used in offices worldwide. In 2015 alone, an estimated 205 billion emails were sent each day worldwide, and that number has climbed to 320 billion emails daily in 2021 (The Radicati Group, 2017). As more people come online, the number will undoubtedly skyrocket, meaning that 24/7 availability and constant interruptions at work and home have become a way of life for remote workers with no real relief in sight.

The lack of workplace privacy is also becoming a significant source of stress. Since workers use workplace computers and networks, their work can be closely monitored in ways that were never possible. That means that even casual viewing of non-work websites can be banned, with many workplaces placing restrictions on internet use, even during off-work hours. Time-and-motion software applications are also becoming increasingly popular, with workers being monitored for "unproductive" computer use and encouraged to use digital devices more efficiently to maximize profit for companies.

Naturally enough, this also means having workers respond to emails and texts from managers as quickly as possible.

To give you an idea about how pervasive this problem has become, a 2013 study looking at information collected by the Android app Locket showed that the 150,000 users in the study checked their phones an average of 110 times a day (Hu, 2013). Granted, some of the reasons users gave for checking their phones included checking the time or looking at photos, but it still highlighted how much they depended on their phones daily.

About three-quarters of the users also unlocked their phones and actively used them during prime evening hours between five and eight p.m. Since these peak evening hours are also prime family time, this constant usage also suggests a significant conflict between work and family life with all the stress and emotional tension that comes with it.

Regular checking of emails, phone texts, etc., have become essential to daily work life. This is due to the proliferation of email notifications, instant messages, task reminders, message reminders, and other interruptions, all delivered by smartphones and tablets that constantly beep, buzz, blink, or (if you're noise-conscious) vibrate. Given the constant need to stay in contact, these interruptions have seriously impacted work productivity, with an estimated two hours a day being lost to digital interruptions.

Even worse, workers are also expected to multitask by handling different streams of information, both internal and external, using smartphone and computer applications such as collaborative software. All of this leads to workers regularly experiencing digital overwhelm since they take in more information than they can safely handle or use efficiently. As a result, not only do they regularly make mistakes and have difficulty meeting production goals but they are also forced to work faster to cope with this influx of new information. This has given rise to new terms such as "information fatigue" and "data fog" to describe what workers regularly experience. For example, even as early as 2005, an international survey of about 8,000 managers showed that one in four executives at large companies felt that their voice and email were more than they could manage. Additionally, nearly half of them spent much of their time on communications that they did not feel were useful for their work (Mandel, 2005).

So, what are the psychological consequences of digital overwhelm in the workplace and home (assuming there is an actual difference anymore)? And how can we cope with the general unhappiness this digital overwhelm can cause the people we care about most and ourselves? To help you understand how digital overwhelm or technostress can be undermining our mental and physical health, let me provide you with a quick overview of stress and what it can do to us.

Understanding Stress

Though everyone knows what you mean when you talk about "being stressed" or "being stressed out", it is still essential to understand stress. Most medical and psychological textbooks describe stress as what happens whenever people are in a threatening situation that exceeds their inner capacity and resources to cope with that stress.

According to stress pioneer Hans Selye, our ability to handle stress occurs in three basic stages: general adaptation syndrome. Ordinarily, our bodies are in a normal state of balance known as *homeostasis*. But, when we encounter a stressful event, we enter what Selye called the alarm reaction stage, in which our body mobilizes to counter the stress. We are basically designed by evolution to respond to threats with a "fight or flight" response in which our bodies prepare us to protect ourselves. As a result, different physiological mechanisms are activated, leading to an increased heart rate, more rapid breathing, the release of cortisol (a stress hormone) into our bloodstream to provide more energy, and a generalized state of arousal.

Once the initial shock wears off, your body will begin trying to restore that original balance. Your heart rate will subside a little, your breathing will slow down, your blood pressure will get back under control, and your condition will stabilize. This is known as the resistance stage, and one of two things will happen: either that initial stressful event will have passed, and you will return to normal, or else your body will adapt, and you will stay on high alert for as long as possible. Though you will feel more under control, your body is still responding to stress behind the scenes. That means your blood pressure will be higher than usual, and your adrenal glands will still release elevated cortisol levels into your bloodstream. While you're in this resistance stage, you will function as close to normal as possible except that you will be more irritable, you will be easily frustrated, you will have trouble sleeping, and your concentration will be affected as well. If this is starting to sound familiar to you, just wait.

If the resistance stage goes on for too long, then your body will end up draining all your mental and physical resources. You will start feeling that things are hopeless, you will become exhausted, burnt-out, more depressed, and you will become even more vulnerable to whatever other stress you might encounter. This stage is the exhaustion stage and, the longer it continues, the more damage it can do to your physical and mental health. This damage includes compromising your immune system leaving you much more susceptible to infections and increased risk of heart disease, cancer, stroke, diabetes, and a host of other conditions.

Your body also begins to "age" much faster, and it can reduce your lifespan in the long run. Emotionally, you become a prime risk for burnout. If the original stress remains chronic, you may find yourself resorting to more extreme ways of countering stress, including substance abuse and suicide in many cases.

How Much Stress Can You Handle?

The important thing to remember about stress is that it is non-specific, meaning it can occur for a variety of reasons, both good and bad. Even happy events such as a wedding or the birth of a child can drain your inner resources, and it is the total amount of stress in your life that counts. There is a familiar stress inventory known as the Holmes-Rahe scale (1967), developed by psychiatrists Thomas Holmes and Richard Rahe as part of their research into whether stress contributes to illness. The scale lists a series of life events, both positive and negative, and the relative impact that they can have on the body. According to Holmes and Rahe, too many of these events occurring in a single year can boost the likelihood of developing stress-related problems. At the very top of the scale is "death of a spouse", followed closely by "divorce", "marital separation", "jail term", and "death of a close family member". Even positive events such as "marriage", "retirement", and "pregnancy" are included in the scale. As for work-related events, "fired at work", "business readjustment", and "change in financial state", can also contribute.

But there are also *micro stressors* or "daily hassles", which, while minor in themselves, can add to your overall stress level in time.

If too much stress occurs in too short a time, or if your body is already weakened by existing stress, then health problems can occur. In addition, your capacity for coping with stress can be compromised further as you grow older and are bothered by the usual medical issues that affect middle-aged or senior adults.

In Japan, there is a familiar term, "karoshi" which means "overwork death". This term applies to employees dying of a stroke, heart disease, suicide, or even starvation due to poor nutrition. According to World Health Organization figures, nearly 800,000 karoshi deaths occurred in 2016 alone in Japan and many other Asian countries. While karoshi is mainly considered an Asian problem, the same work-related stress leading to these deaths is becoming an increasing problem in Western countries, especially in this new era of digital overwhelm.

What Can Save Us from Overwhelm?

While this chapter has focused on the negative consequences of digital technology, it is also important to recognize its positive benefits. For example, many problems resulting from digital overwhelm can be improved with a better workplace organization to consider employee mental health. For example, establishing an explicit email policy ensuring that email is only checked at defined times can significantly decrease stress and help promote employee well-being (Kushlev & Dunn, 2015). Also, despite the problems digital technologies can cause with work-life balance, digital technology can also allow greater flexibility in handling job demands.

In many ways, the recent COVID-19 pandemic has shown that technology has been beneficial in helping people sheltering at home to stay socially connected and even work remotely far more than had ever been permitted in the past. In addition, teleconferencing is becoming more acceptable as a means of connecting with business clients and co-workers and as an educational tool with virtual classrooms replacing in-person classes, at least in the short run. To what extent these changes will become permanent once the current pandemic passes remain to be seen. The resulting freedom remote working provides to workers may help offset some of the negative consequences of technostress and digital overwhelm.

Perhaps more importantly, giving people greater control over when and where they access the information they need to carry out work and school assignments can also help reduce stress. Giving users the means to take "time outs" as required can reduce the risk of burnout though that also depends on company culture and the degree of independence workers are allowed.

Finally, companies also need to establish better communication strategies (e.g., not forwarding emails to employees after business hours). By respecting employee home-time and the need for employee mental health, companies can help prevent technostress problems before they begin.

Unfortunately, work-related stress is only part of the problem with digital overwhelm, and there are far too many other demands on our attention from non-work sources. The often unhealthy dependence we have formed on digital media and the need to stay connected with the latest news and internet memes needs to be addressed as well. We will turn to this in later chapters.

Chapter Three

The Myth of Multitasking

We have already discussed distracted driving in a previous chapter, but the consequences can be truly horrific. On March 29, 2017, concerned drivers called police about a white pickup truck seen swerving and speeding down a highway in Texas. One driver had even recorded a video of this reckless behavior on his smartphone. Despite being alerted, police were unable to catch up to the pickup truck before it ran into a small bus carrying fourteen elderly passengers, all churchgoers, of whom thirteen were killed, and the survivor was severely injured. Based on a reconstruction of the accident, one of the deadliest in state history, the pickup truck driver, 20-year-old Jack Young, had lost control of his vehicle and swerved into the bus's lane resulting in a head-on collision. Young, one of the survivors, admitted that he had been texting while driving at the time of the crash.

In Uvalde County, Texas court sentenced him to 55 years in prison.

There is really no such thing as human multitasking. Though we like to think of ourselves as thinking machines able to carry out two or three important tasks at once, the reality is very different. Yes, you can talk on the phone or listen to music while driving, but splitting your attention means that your ability to respond to task demands will be compromised, at least to some extent.

Understanding Human Multitasking

When you think you are multitasking, what you are doing is switching your attention between different tasks and, if you are good at it, that might allow you to complete the various tasks reasonably well. Since we tend to think of our brains as computers, it becomes easy to believe that we can do the same multitasking that computers seem to do so effortlessly. But, unfortunately, while computers can have multiple processing cores for seamless parallel processing, our biological brains do not have the same multiple architectures.

Since the 1960s, cognitive scientists have studied human multitasking and identified some fundamental limitations to our ability to attend to different tasks at once. Essentially, when we are presented with two competing stimuli (such as checking texts while driving a car), there is a *refractory period* causing our response to one task to be slower because we are still processing that other task.

In one study looking at multitasking, research subjects were asked to tap a specific letter on a keyboard with their right index finger whenever a green light appeared (task one). At the same time, they were also required to push another letter with their left index finger if one digit was displayed while tapping another letter with their left middle finger if another digit was displayed (task 2). When the time needed to respond to the two tasks changed, e.g., 150 milliseconds on one and 1000 milliseconds on the other, the time necessary to complete the second task became much longer, and more errors were made (Pashler, 1994).

Another study had respondents listening on headphones as they were presented a series of numbers and asked whether a number they heard was the same as one they heard one, two, or three places earlier (by pressing "c" for yes or "z" for no on a keyboard with their left hand). The second task involved respondents using their right hand to keep a screen cursor inside a small circular target as it moved around a blue track. Though participants had no trouble with these tasks when carrying them out separately, they had much more difficulty when the two tasks were merged into a single trial. While they still did well on the first task (auditory), their performance on the visual tracking task became steadily worse as the auditory task became more difficult. Also, when asked beforehand how well they thought they would do on this distraction task, even those participants who had the poorest performance thought they would do well (Finley, et al., 2014).

Multitasking in Real Life

If you thought that laboratory studies like this do not necessarily apply to real-life scenarios, such as listening to music while driving, consider the problems faced by air traffic controllers. Though all controllers undergo extensive training before being certified to work in an air traffic tower, they multitask in ways few of us can even imagine. That includes controlling the flight paths of planes, big and small, talking with pilots, responding to air emergencies, and preventing aircraft collisions continuously. Unfortunately, that makes them textbook examples of the disasters that could occur due to even momentary distraction. Yes, major collisions have occurred due to towers being inadequately staffed, staff becoming fatigued by working long hours, staff mismanaging air traffic, or failing to communicate properly with pilots. While air traffic control accidents are becoming rarer thanks to modernized control systems to prevent accidents, errors still occur. In addition, the growing demand for more air towers and air traffic crews may lead to more accidents in the future.

What is the Magic Number?

The main problem with human multitasking is, while we can take in enormous amounts of sensory information that makes it seem as if we can attend to many different things at once, we are often unable to process all that information at once. In a series of classic experiments, cognitive scientist George Armitage Miller determined that our brain's central processor had a basic limit to the amount of information people can attend to at the same time. One example he gave dealt with memory span, or how long a list of items (numbers, letters, or words) we could reliably repeat back after that list is presented to us. Miller concluded that the average young person could only recall seven digits or so, and it was essentially the same for any item list.

Miller also examined how people performed on absolute judgment tasks testing how people responded to different stimuli (to different musical tones, for example). He found that test subjects could only respond to four or eight different alternatives before they started making serious errors.

Based on his findings, in 1956 Miller wrote the classic research paper, "The Magical Number Seven, Plus or Minus Two: Some Limits on Our Capacity for Processing Information". With this, one of the most influential papers in psychology's history, Miller helped lay the groundwork for cognitive psychology and demonstrated the peculiarities of human mental functioning.

Later, researchers added to Miller's research by introducing the concept of working memory, or the short-term storage system we use to retain information temporarily so we can use it for cognitive tasks. According to one prominent model, working memory is made up of different components:

- The central executive, which controls attention and coordinates all the other working memory systems (basically acting as a supervisor over other systems to keep them functioning).
- The phonological loop, which stores language-based information (such as retaining a phone number after having heard it for the first time).
- The visuospatial scratchpad, which stores visual and spatial information (like remembering the route to a place you have seen for the first time)
- The episodic buffer, which links information across different domains to contain short-term memories before passing them on to long-term storage. (Basically linking together different short-term memories before sending them on to be stored long-term).

When it comes to multitasking, working memory acts as a "bottleneck" that limits the amount of information we can process at any given time. Though many people think they are multitasking, what they are doing is alternating between different tasks and, as a result, will typically take much longer and be more prone to error than if they had done these tasks separately.

What usually happens when we multitask is that we prioritize the different tasks we are working on and devote most of our attention to that task that appears most important at the time. With driving, for example, we usually reserve most of our attention to the driving itself unless something calls our attention to another task (like needing to change the station on the radio). Then we are forced to try to keep driving while adjusting the radio and, if something unexpected happens, our reaction time is slowed as a result.

Though it might be possible to *train* the brain to multitask, at least to some extent, that is much harder than you might think. People can be taught to process information more quickly, but that cognitive bottleneck is still there, and errors become inevitable when the different tasks become too complex. Furthermore, how well we can multitask is also affected by conflicting demands by other tasks, so you are forced to prioritize how you respond as a result.

The Spider Model and You

A useful cognitive model, primarily developed to explain distracted driving, can apply to any other occasion when you are forced to multitask. It mainly deals with the situational awareness that is always necessary when you risk being distracted. Known as SPIDER for short, it stands for:

(S)canning for signs of potential threats. Scanning the forward road for potential threats is a must for drivers, but they also need to be aware of any visual blind spots. But even something as basic as checking a rear-view mirror can reduce attention, however briefly. Other frequent multitaskers such as air-traffic controllers and surgeons need to scan constantly as well.

(P)redicting potential threats if they are not visible. Along with visual scanning, multitaskers also need to pay special attention to potential threats they know may be present, based on experience. For drivers, that means watching for someone backing out of a driveway or oncoming traffic hidden by a large truck, etc. That usually means becoming more alert to avoid problems before they develop.

(I)dentifying threats as they occur. This is likely where the most significant chance for making errors can occur. You cannot respond to a threat unless you identify it as one, and if you are distracted for any reason, identification may come too late. Research into distracted driving shows that drivers who are carrying out a secondary task, such as reading a text message on the phone, are prone to inattentional blindness, which prevents them from processing what comes into their field of view. Experiments using eye-tracking to measure attention showed that drives talking on their cell phone were 50 % less likely to recognize safety-critical items in their visual field (including pedestrians, parked cars, oncoming vehicles, etc.) than they would otherwise (Strayer et al., 2003). And the more attention the secondary task demands (such as with a phone call or text message delivering bad news), the worse the inattentional blindness becomes. Though most drivers think they are good at "compartmentalizing" their brains so they can handle both tasks at once, they are often wrong, and the danger of inattentional blindness is very real.

(D)eciding if you need to act and how to do it. Being able to make decisions quickly is critical in tasks such as driving. For example, when deciding to change lanes or make a left turn with oncoming traffic, drivers need to consider traffic conditions to ensure they can do this safely. But, when drivers are distracted, even by a hands-free phone, it becomes far too easy to make mistakes like misjudging the size of a traffic gap or the speed of an oncoming vehicle, especially in bad weather conditions or if the road is wet. The more divided your attention, the greater the risk of a serious crash.

(E)xecuting appropriate (R)esponses. Once that decision is made, reaction time becomes critically important. And so, when something happens that requires a fast response (such as an animal or a child running across the road), distracted drivers are not going to respond as quickly as they otherwise might. The more distracted a driver is (for example, talking on the phone or dealing with traffic conditions), the more sluggish that driver's braking speed will be.

Though it is easy to think that the SPIDER model only relates to driving, the need for situation awareness can apply wherever or whenever you face the potential of an accident or injury. This could happen at work, when walking in unfamiliar neighborhoods, or even in the privacy of your own home. The National Safety Council has identified "distracted walking" as a significant safety threat, with more than 11,000 injuries occurring between 2000 and 2011 resulting from cell-phone use while walking. Phone distractions can result in people tripping, crossing roads unsafely, or walking into objects such as street signs, doors, or walls. Though many of these injuries can also occur in the workplace, they are harder to track as most injured workers may not want to admit to being distracted by phone use.

And at least half of those distracted walking injuries occur right in the home. The risk of tripping over some furniture, slipping in the shower, or being injured while doing a home repair task, rises sharply when people are distracted by a cell phone or other digital device. Because people think they are in a safe place, they may be less likely to be cautious, and in return the more distracted they are going to be by a phone conversation, watching a video, or texting.

Is Automation the Answer?

With the number of accidents being regularly linked to distracted driving (or walking, for that matter), it is hardly surprising that car and home automation have become multibillion-dollar industries. Along with the development of "smart cars" that relieve drivers of many of the tasks involved in avoiding collisions, we are also seeing a proliferation in "smart home" devices allowing digital devices to be controlled by voice alone.

Though truly autonomous cars are still decades away (despite the claims of various pundits who might say otherwise), semi-autonomous vehicles are already on the road offering such functions as adaptive cruise control, collision avoidance, lane centering, etc. By controlling car speed and steering, these cars take much of the risk out of the hands of human drivers who need only act when the car systems fail (such as in poor road conditions or lane markers beginning to fade). How autonomous cars will be in five to ten years remains to be seen.

But would semi-autonomous cars really solve the problem of distracted driving? Probably not considering how poor humans are at tasks involving continuous monitoring, which drivers would still be required to do to ensure their semi-automatic cars do not run into problems. Research into maritime and aviation operations (e.g., naval personnel watching radar screens or aircrews watching instrument panels in mid-flight) suggests that humans have a major problem staying focused for long periods of time due to boredom or because they are understimulated. This brings us to a somewhat underappreciated aspect of human psychology known as the Yerkes-Dodson Law. First proposed by psychologists Robert Yerkes (pronounced YERK-ees) and John D. Dodson in 1908, this law was based on their research into the relationship between how well people perform on different tasks and mental arousal, or the extent to which the brain is stimulated.

What Yerkes and Dodson found was that there was an *inverted U-curve* defining this relationship. As you can see from the diagram below, performing well on a specific task (such as driving) means that your brain needs to be optimally stimulated. If your brain is *under-stimulated* (for example, you are bored or tired), your performance will suffer, but if it is *overstimulated* (due to being overly excited or frightened), your performance suffers as well.

When it comes to driving long distances, for example, people can often slip into an altered state of consciousness, if not falling asleep altogether, because their brains are not sufficiently stimulated to keep them alert at the wheel. A 2011 research study tested how well people could drive at differing levels of automation (Dong et al., 2011). The study had participants drive a simulated vehicle under three conditions: manual driving, regular cruise control (the system controls the speed but not the distance to the forward vehicle), and adaptive cruise control (the system automatically controls the speed while maintaining a safe distance to the forward vehicle). Though automatic systems made driving easier, drivers tended to be slower to react to changing road conditions requiring them to take full control of their vehicles. This usually happened because their brains were not as aroused as under the manual driving condition. Though there has been less research on other forms of automation, the same problem applies, which means that the issue of distracted driving or walking still needs to be solved.

As we have seen in this chapter, humans are not the best at multitasking, and the more distracted you are by a secondary task, the more likely you are to make mistakes at your main task. Moreover, since we can only attend to a limited amount of information at any given time, we must switch our attention between tasks, often with tragic results. In an era of digital overwhelm, coming to terms with constant distractions and the need to shift attention as unexpected interruptions occur seems to be the price we must pay for being increasingly connected with the world around us. Though we can learn to adapt, at least to some extent, finding relief from this constant need to multitask and staying focused on critical tasks, not to mention avoiding errors, is a problem yet to be solved.

Chapter Four

Digital Distractions

For as long as television has existed, parents and teachers have worried about the impact of too much television-watching on their children. Along with worrying about the thousands of television deaths the average child witnessed over time, parents also worried about how watching television often crowded out healthier alternatives such as spending quality time with friends or family. But how much worse has the problem become with the proliferation of digital devices children have access to these days? All of which has led to a sharp rise in time spent with their eyes glued to the screen.

This is not a problem for children alone though much of the research looking at the effect of total screen time on mental and emotional development seems to focus primarily on children and adolescents. However, a sobering 2017 study suggests that even toddlers can be adversely affected by the constant interruptions caused by smartphone use by their parents.

The study (Reed, et al., 2017) recruited forty-four mothers and their two-year-old children and had each mother-child dyad complete two trials during which they taught their child one of two invented words. The two words were blicking (which was meant to be the same as bouncing) and frepping (shaking) using a gender-neutral doll. The word learning was uninterrupted during one trial, but the other trial involved a 30-second telephone call in the middle of the word learning.

During the experimental condition in which the mother received a telephone call, most mothers just shifted their attention away from their child to answer the call. Some mothers prepared their children for the interruption with phrases such as "Hold on, sweetheart, Mama's getting a phone call." When the phone conversation occurred, toddlers typically responded either by waiting patiently for their mothers to resume talking to them or wandering away searching for a new diversion. After the call was over, the mothers turned to their children and continued teaching them the new word. The order of the two trials was randomly varied for mother-child pairs, and each child was assessed following the trial to see how well they had learned the new word.

You probably won't be too shocked to learn that the toddlers were far more likely to learn the invented words during the uninterrupted condition than during the condition which was interrupted by the phone call. This difference appears to be due primarily to the quality of the communication between mothers and their children. While mothers generally used the invented words more often in the interrupted condition rather than the control condition (24 times vs 20 times), toddlers in the control condition still learned better.

To explain these findings, the researchers argued that children in their first two or three years of life are especially sensitive to the verbal and non-verbal cues that mothers and other caregivers give off while communicating. That means that even supposedly "harmless" disruptions such as answering a smartphone can have an impact on emotional and language development.

And the risk of constant digital disruptions can have even more of an impact as children grow older. In an era of increasingly affordable digital devices, more parents than ever are splurging to ensure that their children have access to the latest gadgets. As a result, not only are children getting their own smartphones, often before reaching their teen years, but they are also getting video games, their own computers to do homework and surf the Internet, and even flat-screen televisions for them to enjoy in their own bedrooms. All of which can have a serious impact on their mental and emotional health.

Take sleep, for example. It is suggested that an infant needs from twelve to sixteen hours of sleep, while children aged thirteen and over need around eight to ten hours. Though the amount of sleep that a child needs drops over time, not getting that sleep will have a major effect on a child's ability to stay awake and alert during the day (especially in school).

A child's natural sleep schedule can be easily thrown off by digital devices such as smartphones and tablets, which brings us to melatonin, a hormone produced by the pineal gland in the brain. Because of how our bodies evolved, we have a natural circadian rhythm (a 24-hour cycle that alternates in tune with our exposure to light. For most of human history (and well before), our circadian rhythm was in tune with the typical day-night cycle, with melatonin levels slowly increasing as it became darker.

Unfortunately, the rise of artificial light in the past two centuries has had an adverse effect on our regular sleep cycles. Along with street lighting, all homes are now equipped with electric lights and, more recently, with television sets that can play havoc with our regular sleep schedule.

All of which brings us back to children and adolescents, many of whom have digital devices right in their bedrooms, which can often cost them valuable sleep time. According to sleep experts, digital devices such as smartphones, tablets, video games, and computers all have screens that emit a "blue light" that can suppress the natural buildup of melatonin. This reduces the number of hours of sleep a child is able to get at night, and it can also affect the quality of the sleep that they do get. The result is that they are much drowsier during the day, undermining their ability to pay attention in school and learn properly. For that matter, adults are increasingly having the same problem due to the distractions coming from digital devices.

Some companies are trying to combat this problem. One of these companies is Apple, introducing a "Night Shift" feature in its products. This feature basically uses the iPhone or iPad clock and geolocation to automatically adjust the colors in the display towards the "warmer" end of the spectrum. Then, in the morning, the display automatically returns to normal, hopefully allowing for a good night's sleep. Though there is no equivalent feature for Android devices yet, free apps are already available, which work similarly.

Still, features like this are likely not enough to solve the blue-light problems, especially since any source of light penetrating through eyelids is enough to disrupt melatonin production (which is why workers on the night shift have so much trouble sleeping during the day). As a result, experts advise against watching television or using any digital device for at least thirty minutes before going to sleep.

However, this is often a hard rule to follow. Especially for young people with televisions or other possible distractions right in their own bedrooms, posing an ever-present temptation to "tire themselves out" digitally if they are having trouble falling asleep. And so, the problem of losing sleep becomes even harder to solve.

Another problem is the unexpected "pings" or ring tones if someone sends an email message or tries to phone after someone is already asleep. Though many people set their phones to vibrate or shut off the notification feature on their devices at night, many don't, and few of us have the discipline not to reach for that device to see what someone is saying. This brings us to the other reason why so many of us are reluctant to stay digitally disconnected for long, the FOMO factor.

Learning about FOMO

Afraid you will miss out on some hot new meme, some important news, or the chance of getting into something important or rewarding? Of course, you are. This fear brings us to FOMO, short for "Fear of Missing Out", and it is becoming ever more essential in this digital age. FOMO was formally defined as "a pervasive apprehension that others might be having rewarding experiences from which one is absent...characterized by the desire to stay continually connected with what others are doing". It highlights the anxiety most social media users experience over potentially missing out on something important or fun.

Granted, the need to stay informed has an ancient history, with villagers eagerly asking travelers for news from the next town or town criers announcing the latest news at the top of their lungs. Moreover, even the popularity of the first printing presses was largely driven by the need to pass on information with much more accuracy than the old word-of-mouth system. For that matter, FOMO seems to be universal across cultures. As one example, the word kiasu originating from the Hokkien (Chinese) dialect is generally translated as the "fear of missing out" or" the fear of losing out to someone else", and this is hardly unique.

The rise of the Internet and social media imposes far more challenges than ever before. Not only are we bombarded with news, memes, social media posts, and notifications about upcoming events, but constantly keeping up with all of them becomes impossible. Among young people especially, to a large extent, this fear of missing out drives their need to stay online as much as they can. While survey studies from 2011-2012 already showed that three-quarters of all young people sampled reported feeling uneasy about missing out on what their age peers were doing, our growing dependence on digital devices has likely pushed this figure even higher.

While most available research has focused mainly on how FOMO affects social media use, biomedical studies have already identified mental health problems linked to FOMO, including increased depression and social anxiety. For young people, much of their social identity and self-esteem stems from how they are viewed by others, particularly peers their own age. News about positive and fun things happening to other people often triggers a sense of inadequacy, especially if this news makes their own lives seem less interesting as a result. Young people who are already feeling isolated (particularly given the effects of the recent pandemic), may feel less popular or that they are losing out on the exciting things happening to friends or acquaintances on social media.

FOMO has also been directly linked to less success with face-to-face relationships, poorer academic performance, and reduced motivation, to name just a few psychological issues studied. For example, a 2016 study examined the associations between social media use, FOMO, and different mental and physical health outcomes for a large sample of U.S. university students. The results showed that people with a greater fear of missing out experienced more physical symptoms (including headaches, shortness of breath, sore throat, etc.), more depressive symptoms, and less mindful awareness of their mental and physical state. Moreover, these relationships still apply even when the researchers account for the participants' total time on social networks. This indicates that these relationships are essential above and beyond social media use alone (Baker, et al., 2017).

Though much more research needs to be done, the FOMO problem is not likely to go away anytime soon. If anything, it will likely become even worse, considering how interconnected the entire world has come to be and the essential role that internet use plays in how people of all ages live their lives.

Digital Distractions in the Home

According to a new report released by the Gonski Institute for Education at the University of New South Wales in Sydney, Australia, parents are more worried than ever about their children's digital habits (Graham & Sahlberg, 2021). Though digital devices are great for helping parents keep track of their children's whereabouts and always stay in contact with them, the parents in the study were also aware that those devices had a dark side.

The study, titled Growing Up Digital Australia, is part of an international research effort by universities from multiple countries to investigate how digital media and technologies impact children's wellbeing, health, and eventually learning at school. Growing Up Digital Australia collected data about more than 5,000 children across Australia through comprehensive interviews with thousands of parents, grandparents, and caregivers for their research.

According to the study, nine out of ten parents reported feeling that digital devices negatively distracted their own lives. At the same time, 83% also viewed their children as being negatively distracted. "Parents think that digital media and technologies have a dual power of offering children both benefits and drawbacks," said Professor Pasi Sahlberg, Deputy Director of the Gonski Institute for Education, in a media interview about the study. "Hence, we need smart solutions to address these complex challenges towards sustainable digital wellness for our youth."

That same study also found that about a third of families regularly allowed their children to use their digital devices after bedtime every single day. Also, 60% of children who struggle in school typically sleep with digital gadgets in their bedrooms. There were also socioeconomic differences, with children from lower-income households being most at risk by digital distractions since their parents were less likely to monitor their children's screen-time or to believe that it adversely affected their development.

They likely had reason to be concerned since four out of five of the children in the study owned at least one screen-based device, with an average of 3.3 devices per child. Since personal ownership of a digital device began as early as four in many cases, almost all the children in the study had no real experience of a world that didn't include the technology they took for granted.

Overall, the parents in the study agreed that digital distractions often got in the way of children doing other things they considered to be healthier. For example, about 73% of parents felt digital activities caused children to be less physically active, have a reduced attention span (62%), be less creative, and be less likely to spend time with families. Granted, parents also recognized positive aspects of digital technology, which they credited with improving their children's mathematical and reading ability.

When it came to actual solutions for the effects of digital distraction on children, parents acknowledged that they were part of the problem, with 90% of them admitting to being digitally distracted themselves. Most parents also felt that the situation was worsening, especially since they had little actual control over their children's viewing habits. Even for parents who "got tough" and confiscated the digital devices their children used to force a digital "time-out", the negative consequences, including significant depression in many children, often appeared to make the problem worse.

The same Growing Up Digital study also interviewed nearly two thousand teachers across Australia to measure their concerns about the impact of digital distractions on the children they taught. About 84 % of teachers stated that the distractions provided by digital devices were a growing problem in classrooms. As a result, not only were a large percentage of children coming to school visibly tired and with poorer attention spans, but incomplete homework assignments were becoming more of a problem for many of them.

Perhaps not coincidentally, cyberbullying and online harassment was also becoming much more common. Of the teachers surveyed, one in three reported having dealt with ten or more incidents of cyberbullying or harassment in the previous five years. Over 90 % of teachers also stated that the number of children with psychological, social, and behavioral issues had risen sharply over the past five years. They also felt that children showed much less empathy and were much less physically active overall. As for the positive benefits of digital technology, teachers seem to be a little more mixed, with only 43% feeling that the devices enhanced teaching and learning. While schools are trying to rein in digital use during class time, including banning the use of smartphones and other devices in class, this is largely a losing battle, at least for now.

When it came to their own digital use, the teachers and principals surveyed seemed to report the same problems with digital distractions that parents did. Younger teachers (under the age of twenty-five) seem much more aware of the issues posed by digital technology. In fact, up to 61 % of these younger teachers admitted to being digital addicts themselves, making them all too aware of the problems this technology posed for an entire generation of children and adolescents. While most schools have "get tough" policies when it comes to digital use in schools, including requiring phones to be handed in to teachers before class or else only allowing students to use their devices during recess or lunch, these policies do nothing to curb digital use at home.

These problems are hardly limited to Australia. Growing Up Digital studies in other parts of the world, including the United States and Canada, are reporting similar trends. If anything, the digital distraction has become even more severe given the recent pandemic and the resulting lockdowns. After the use of virtual classrooms and children returning to school, their dependence on digital devices seems more ingrained than ever.

In this chapter, we have covered some of the problems digital distractions pose for children and adolescents and hints about what effect this growing dependence on digital technology may have as these children grow into adults. In a real sense, parents and teachers have little experience dealing with issues such as FOMO, cyberbullying, online harassment, or dealing with predators. This lack of experience means they often feel helpless when trying to help children control their digital use. However, this is rapidly becoming a problem for people of all ages, especially with the rise of the Attention Economy. More on that in the next chapter.

Chapter Five

Everything's Fighting for Your Attention

Hearing the phone ring in the middle of the night is never a good thing. If you happen to be asleep at the time, you are likely to feel groggy as you come to terms with the fact that anyone calling you so late is unlikely to be delivering good news. Even worse, imagine this is in the bad old days before Caller ID or answering services, so you have no idea who is on the other end of the line or what they want. You are then left with the choice of either letting the phone ring or not. If you ignored it, the phone would stop before long though, if it is urgent, then whoever it is will likely phone back before long. Alternatively, you can reach over to pick up the phone and hope that the conversation will not leave you too upset to get back to sleep afterward. And that was the reality of life before the rise of digital devices.

However, now the world is a very different place. While you can still get that late-night phone call, there is a Caller ID to weed out the urgent callers from the wrong numbers and other frivolous calls that can occur. For that matter, you might set your smartphone to silent or vibrate, so you can enjoy a good night's sleep, secure in knowing that whoever is calling will leave a message (usually).

Unfortunately, shutting out the world is becoming harder to do. Not only do smartphones provide different ringtones for different people in your life, but more computer applications than ever now provide "push" notifications that alert you about even the most trivial developments. That includes alerting you that you have a new email or text message, that a particular app has a new update that you must have (assuming the app doesn't just install it automatically), or notifying you about the latest "big savings" offer by assorted sales sites that you *shouldn't* miss. However, this is just the tip of the iceberg when it comes to the "Attention Economy", and what this likely means for the future.

Understanding the Attention Economy

First described by psychologist and author Herbert Simon back in the 1970s, the central problem of a world rich in information was that it created an *attention scarcity* since human brains were limited in how much data they could pay attention to at any time. As a result, information overload remains an ongoing problem for users of all ages. It also means that the countless content producers, including large corporations, bloggers, information sites, and social media posters need to *compete* for the average user's attention.

The result of this competition is an attention economy, which has transformed our lives more than anyone could have predicted even a decade ago. The commercialization of the Internet now means that we are regularly besieged by advertisements, notifications, personalized news feeds, Buzzfeed-style headlines, fake news, public service announcements, etc. All the organizations providing this content rely heavily on the latest research findings in media and cognitive psychology to shape their message in the most attractive way possible. They also rely on mass A/B testing (experimental research using different versions of the same message to see which is more effective) to draw people in to buy their product.

An entire industry is now dedicated to ensuring the best possible coverage for content, with new terms such as "click-through rates" and "daily active users" to describe different ways of measuring their success. In addition, virtually every new marketing or business school graduate now receives training in "search engine optimization (SEO)" to learn different ways of tweaking content to ensure that it is at the top of any web search. Google and other search engine companies offer specialized analysis services that speed up the SEO process and ensure maximum saturation of online markets.

But it isn't just companies that are struggling for our limited attention. Video sites such as YouTube and Tik Tok allow virtually anyone with a video camera (or only a smartphone) to post videos and attract viewers. There are also other sites such as Reddit, Instagram, Facebook. Twitter, etc., all designed to draw in viewers as they share new memes, old memes, blog posts, podcasts, or whatever other content they might want to share. Along with the great dream of having content "go viral", there are more opportunities than ever for people to make money from the people following their efforts.

For now, at least, the attention economy is primarily controlled by five companies:

- Meta, which owns Facebook, Instagram, WhatsApp, Oculus VR and many related sites and apps

- Alphabet (the latest incarnation of Google, which owns Google Search, Twitter, and YouTube, among other concerns)
- Tencent, ByteDance, and Sina Corporation, all of which are Chinese companies dominating the China market and making inroads into Western markets with TikTok and other social media sites

Still, with more than five billion web users (a figure that is rising steadily), and nearly two billion websites (also rising fast), there are sites to accommodate a vast range of interests, as well as a thriving "Dark Net" for those whose interests are frankly illegal or unethical.

There are also spammers sending out multiple unsolicited email, text, phone, or video ads. Though most spam messages are sent out for the sole purpose of generating interest in various products, many of them also distribute "malware" (harmful software such as viruses and Trojan Horses). These harmful apps, ranging from the simple to the complex, are designed to take over a computer to steal financial information or send harmful software to other systems. And as a result, we are also besieged by advertisements for companies offering software to protect us from malware and unwanted ads.

Make no mistake about the attention economy; its sole currency is the amount of attention that content producers can attract, whether in the number of clicks that a post can bring in or how much advertisement they can sell. You are targeted whenever you turn on your digital device, and the ones targeting you will do whatever it takes to get your attention. All too frequently, that means relying on inflammatory and often outrageous statements about current news events, celebrities in the news, and media stories intended to arouse fear, outrage, sympathy, pity, or simply a chance to coo at the latest videos of cute babies, puppies, etc.

We can see grim examples of this with virtually any controversial issue you can name, including purveyors of misinformation selling the latest health cure. During the COVID-19 pandemic, fears about vaccination produced a ready-made market for assorted "cures" as well as horror stories about the dangers of novel vaccines. Along with websites intended to draw in potential customers and recruit new believers, posts denouncing the Center for Disease Control and medical authorities such as Dr. Anthony Fauci were repeatedly villainized because that was what many people wanted to believe.

So, how can we handle all this traffic, not to mention the constant notifications, whether in the form of musical tones or popup notes that can distract you no matter what you happen to be doing at the time? For that matter, is it possible for us to escape from digital overwhelm, or are we too addicted to the Internet to escape from its pull? More on that in the next section.

How Widespread is Social Media Addiction?

In many ways, social media is virtually universal. As of July 20, there were an estimated 4 billion social media users, half of them on Facebook alone. Indeed, there is no disputing that social media can be a force for good, with countless users relying on it to make new friends and staying in touch with old ones no matter how far away they happen to be. Granted, social media sites such as Facebook and Twitter can be among the worst offenders for "push" notifications alerting users about new posts or feedback about changes to friendship networks, how popular their posts have been, etc.

But what about the emotional impact too much social media use can have, especially when you consider the enormous number of research studies that came out in the past twenty years. Terms like "Facebook depression," "Facebook anxiety," and "social media depression" introduced in the past two decades highlight how widespread the impact of mental health issues linked to social media can be.

All of which brings us to the controversial topic of social media addiction. Researchers have long recognized that people can form a psychological dependence on behaviors such as gambling, stress eating, and hair-pulling in the same way they can become dependent on certain drugs.

Researchers are largely divided on whether people can become addicted to social media since there is no commonly accepted definition. Though "Internet Gaming Disorder" has been included in the latest version of the Diagnostic and Statistical Manual of Mental Disorders (DSM-5), there is nothing equivalent for those who are addicted to internet use.

Several psychometric tests, which are designed to measure problem behavior in internet users, have been developed. The most popular one is the Bergen Facebook Addiction Scale (BFAS, 2015). This is an 18-item scale measuring different aspects of internet addiction, including items measuring relapse, withdrawal, and mood effects. The BFAS has been used worldwide on research participants of all ages. Other versions adapted to social media use include items such as: "How often in the past year have you felt an urge to use social media more and more".

A 2021 study examining BFAS scores in 63 independent samples across 32 nations showed that social media addiction's actual prevalence varies widely depending on cultural differences and how rigidly research participants are classified (Cheng et al, 2021). In North America, the average prevalence rate for social media addiction was around 15 % compared to 37 % in Africa and 29 % in the Middle East.

The study also shows that younger people appear much more vulnerable to social media addiction than older adults, primarily because they were introduced to it at a much younger age and are more comfortable with communicating that way. Still, the recent pandemic has worsened addiction symptoms for people of all ages, leading to problems such as reduced work productivity, and lower life satisfaction.

How Can Digital Distractions Be Handled?

Those same libraries that are often seen as largely obsolete in an era of digital books and online internet searches seem to have gained new importance for college students as a sanctuary for studying away from digital distractions. For example, an interesting study by the Project Information Library at the University of Washington shows libraries to be especially important for students at "crunch time" while preparing for exams (Wojcik, 2012).

The researchers conducted hundreds of interviews with students on ten different college or university campuses during the weeks leading up to final exams. While 40 % of those students still used smartphones and laptops, few took any other digital devices. "Most students tended to have cell or smartphones so they could keep in touch as they studied, and then a laptop or library desktop computer for preparing assignments, research, studying and reading," says lead researcher Alison J. Head.

She also noted that few undergraduates interviewed in the libraries spent time playing games, looking at YouTube videos, emailing friends, or "otherwise demonstrating the lack of attention so often attributed to today's students." Instead, the most used computer applications were web browsers for research or word processing programs. "Only 13 percent had Facebook open at the time of the interviews," said Head, and then often as an incentive or reward for finishing their work.

The upshot of the research is that college students seem capable of "dialing down" their technology use as needed. "Students talked about using the library as a refuge," Head reported. "They … lock themselves in a study room where there are no distractions." Many students in the study even reported relying on the library computers since this allowed them to avoid distractions by the applications installed on their home computers.

Despite the popular cliché of young people balancing several different devices and being continually distracted, Head and her fellow researchers suggested that this didn't appear to be the case. "We found students really attempting to manage their devices and strike a balance between scholastic productivity and personal communication," she said.

Despite such encouraging results, not all researchers are quite so optimistic. Research looking at the impact of using smartphones and other digital devices in classrooms consistently demonstrates just how distracting these devices can be. For example, Froese et al. (2012) found that students who participated in active text conversations during a PowerPoint presentation leading up to a quiz had lower quiz scores by an average of 27% compared to students who were not texting during the presentation. For that matter, survey studies indicated that students know that using their personal devices during class splits their attention. McCoy (2013) found that 90% of students indicated not paying attention as one of the three most significant disadvantages to using a digital device in class for purposes not related to the class. In addition, 80% indicated missing instruction as another major disadvantage.

When exploring the reasons why students would use their digital devices during class time knowing about the potential drawbacks, McCoy (2013) also reported that 55 % of students surveyed listed fighting boredom as a primary reason. Though 49 % of the students reported using their devices for classroom-related reasons, including trying to learn more as the lecture unfolded, this still represented a potential distractor that caused them to miss concepts outlined during lectures.

To fight the distractions caused by digital devices, many schools have enacted formal policies banning their use during class time, even to the point of confiscating devices found to violate those policies. There also appears to be a formal system of etiquette that has sprung over the use of digital devices in settings where they are considered inappropriate, such as class lectures and business meetings. Unfortunately, as we will see in the next section, these etiquette systems may become even harder to avoid in the future.

Into the Future and the Internet of Things

Despite the digital intrusions that have become part of our daily lives, the future is likely to be even more hectic with the rise of the Internet of Things (IoT). While artificial intelligence applications such as Amazon Alexa and Google Assistant are already connecting various digital devices with a voice-controlled interface to streamline their use, IoT is expected to have an even more profound effect on our lives.

Imagine smart homes in which your refrigerator, automobile, music center, television, etc., are all part of a single network, each of which can notify you as needed. This includes smart security cameras alerting you of something moving in your yard, smart refrigerators informing you that certain foods or drinks are getting low, cars that warn you that fluid levels need to be topped up, and so forth. The IoT will also revolutionize health care by continuously monitoring seniors or other people with chronic medical needs, including wearable heart monitors and alert systems tied directly into cochlear implants for the hearing impaired.

Automobiles linked into IoT networks will also allow drivers to be notified of any problems at home and work, monitor traffic, keep track of toll collection, and eventually pave the way to self-driving vehicles. IoT applications are also expected to be particularly common in most workplaces considering the sheer range of different industrial and manufacturing uses already being planned.

Though the expanded use of IoT will likely mean a profound change in the way we live and work, it will also mean a sharp increase in the digital distractions people will be expected to cope with over an average day. Researchers are already raising concerns about how the IoT will undermine privacy even more than what we take for granted now (Monteith et al., 2021). Considering that our digital viewing habits are being constantly monitored to provide companies with information about us to make advertisements more effective, IoT networks will undoubtedly help this process. How well will we be able to ignore advertisements specifically tailored to even our most private viewing and buying habits? And how effective will these new digital distractions be in the future as companies continue to make them more addictive?

In this chapter, we have explored many of the issues surrounding digital distractions, including how they change the way we live, learn, work and how they are likely to change us even further in the future. While schools and workplaces are already enacting formal policies to reduce possible distractions, the rise of the Attention Economy, social media addiction, and the Internet of Things seem designed to make this harder than ever before. And then, there is the growing problem of digital clutter and digital hoarding, more on this in the next chapter.

Chapter Six

Digital Clutter and Digital Hoarding

How many tabs are open on your web browser right now? For that matter, how many emails are there in your inbox, and how many pictures, music files, videos, text files, or plain junk is currently on your computer, most of which you are unlikely ever to look at again?

Everyone seems to have a good idea about what constitutes hoarding disorder. According to the DSM-V, it is classified as an obsessive need to accumulate an enormous number of objects ranging from old newspapers to pets in many cases. Though we typically only hear about the extreme cases with people being found buried under piles of old junk in their homes, hoarding disorder is a lot more common than most people think. But is there really such a thing as *digital hoarding*?

As it happens, yes, there is. A 2015 case study represents the first case of digital hoarding behavior reported in the clinical literature (van Bennekom et al., 2015). The case involved a 47-year-old man referred to an outpatient treatment clinic for help in dealing with his compulsive need to take hundreds of digital photographs a day and hoard them, along with other signs of hoarding such as collecting pieces of paper and bike components, which were cluttering his entire house. To keep all his digital photographs, he had four large external hard drives containing the original pictures and another four hard drives to contain the backups. Though he never looked at the images once he collected them, he seemed convinced that they would be valuable in the future and refused to get rid of them.

Since he planned to publish the pictures someday, he spent four to five hours each day arranging his collection and reported feeling frustrated at all the time this required. Along with his photography and picture arranging taking up much of his daily life, it also interfered with other activities, including sleeping.

Not only was this man not married, but he was also unemployed and lived on a disability allowance (he had been diagnosed with autism spectrum disorder and attention deficit disorder years earlier). He also had a family history of hoarding behavior. Though he met the DSM-V criteria for hoarding behavior, the lack of any previous cases of digital hoarding made his case unique. Based on his symptoms, the authors coined the term digital hoarding, which they defined as "the accumulation of digital files to the point of loss of perspective, which eventually results in stress and disorganization." The case study ended with him still undergoing counseling for his hoarding behavior, which continued at that time.

Another extreme example of digital hoarding comes from a 2011 news story by a Florida television station (Anfinsen, 2011). Describing a Fort Lauderdale resident with six computers in his home, the story described him as being incapable of deleting anything from junk emails to unwanted files. Not only did the man react with disbelief at having to delete any of the vast number of files on his systems, but he also insisted that he would simply purchase more computers if he ever needed more memory space. The story also described the phenomenon of "e-hoarding" as being a growing problem for computer users. A local psychologist suggests that the root of such extreme digital hoarding likely stems from hoarders being unable to decide what is essential and what isn't.

While these are extreme cases, virtually everyone who uses digital devices engages in some form of digital hoarding as more and more files continue to accumulate. Granted, this may not seem like much of a problem considering the average hard drive can contain terabytes of information while cloud storage makes virtually limitless storage available for everyone. But that still means the average computer user can accumulate tens of thousands of files that are never deleted because they "might become useful someday."

In a study published in the journal Computers in Human Behavior (Sweeten et al., 2018), a sample of 45 people was questioned about their digital hoarding behavior and their reasons for not deleting unused files. The answers they provided ranged from simple laziness to feeling distressed at the thought of deleting any files they considered potentially useful at some point.

The same research team also developed a Digital Hoarding Questionnaire (DHQ) to measure the extent of digital hoarding as a problem in the workplace. The DHQ is made up of ten questions, scored on a five-point scale, and organized into two sections: Difficulty Deleting and Accumulating. The DHQ questions included "I find it extremely difficult to delete old or unused files, "Deleting certain files would be like deleting a loved one," and "Deleting certain files would be like losing part of myself".

The researchers found that email was a particular concern, with the average inbox containing 102 unread and 331 read emails. "People are very aware that it's a problem, but they're hampered by the way that their organizations typically do things," said lead researcher Nick Neave in a BBC interview (Oakes, 2019). "They've got this flood of emails, and they daren't get rid of them, and things mount up."

Considering that most of the emails are work-related, the people studied often provided valid reasons to hold on to emails and other files, whether needing to keep a record for work purposes or because they are afraid of the consequences of getting rid of files that might be needed someday. But what about the digital clutter that most people accumulate with time? Does this count as digital hoarding or not?

In that same BBC article, two professors from Australia's Monash University described their research interviewing over 800 Australians about their digital hoarding, as well as the emotional problems it tended to cause. They found that digital hoarders often experienced the same stress reported by many physical hoarders, as well as grief at deleting files they think they might need later.

Another professor interviewed, Jo-Ann Oravec of the University of Wisconsin-Whitewater, argued that digital hoarding was not so much about accumulating information as it is about being in control of the data they have collected. Still, when too much data is collected, many people may feel that they are losing that control. "My students tell me it's nausea. It's a sense of disequilibrium when they begin to look through the masses of photos that they have," she said. Nick Neave also agrees that digital clutter may affect people in different ways. "If they get to that point where they've become overwhelmed by the data that they've got, that they can't find things, that things are getting lost... that may indicate that there's some kind of problem."

Is There a Cost to Digital Hoarding?

Leaving aside the psychological costs of digital hoarding, the sheer volume of new data produced each day (an estimated 2.5 quintillion bytes of data) and the need to store it all have environmental costs that are only beginning to be understood. Yes, computer memory and cloud storage systems are relatively cheap, but data use and storage still consume electricity. Along with being used by computers, electrical power is also needed to transmit data across the world. Furthermore, the enormous server farms also depend on electricity to store all this data, and so do the cooling systems keeping the servers operational.

On average, the electricity needed by servers alone is responsible for around two percent of the annual electricity production in the United States. This figure is already more significant than the annual energy costs of most nations. While technological advances may help curb this energy demand, more pessimistic estimates suggest that, by 2030, total energy demands by data networks and services will be greater than twenty percent annually worldwide and rising.

Despite the growing popularity of alternative energy sources, many locations still require burning fossil fuels for electrical production, meaning that the average carbon costs linked to data systems are also rising. But according to the latest annual ClickClean report released by Greenpeace International, many prominent IT companies, such as Facebook, Apple, and Google, have made public commitments to phasing out fossil fuel use in favor of renewable energy. However, many other companies have been slow to follow suit.

Can We Control Digital Hoarding and Cluttering?

In a real sense, it is easy to blame various technology companies for making digital hoarding so affordable and straightforward. With the vast amount of computer memory at the disposal of the average computer user, there is no real problem with keeping virtually every detail of our individual lives on file for decades, whether we will ever need it.

Also, due to the virtual nature of digital hoarding, even extreme hoarders can still avoid many of the problems seen in physical hoarders. They can live seemingly ordinary lives with few visible signs of emotional distress or other mental health issues. Except, of course, for the emotional grief they may feel from trying to keep track of all the different files they might have and the sense of distress that might arise from losing files due to system crashes or other computer problems.

Digital cluttering can likely be seen as a more gentle form of digital hoarding. However, it is far more common and can usually be identified by people seeing too many desktop icons or having memory problems from the sheer number of files on their computers. Mind you, this kind of buildup can occur for other reasons, particularly as new applications add icons to your desktop and take up more memory space. It might be hard to fill up a multi-terabyte hard drive, but hardly impossible.

The most important distinction between digital hoarding and digital clutter is that hoarders intend to hang on to their data due to a fear of losing something important, while clutter piles up because we are either too lazy or too busy to get rid of it. Therefore, digital housekeeping becomes especially important, both in terms of clearing computer space and getting rid of obsolete junk that no longer has any real purpose.

Admittedly, this can often be difficult since every new application you install on your computer will also install an enormous number of mysterious files, which may or may not be necessary for running this new application. Even your operating system will do this, and you might find that wiping a specific file might make your computer go wonky or even shut down completely (it happens more often than you might think). Then there are the text, video, audio, or picture files that you downloaded long ago and which you haven't looked at in years. Just list your different files in File Explorer or some equivalent application to tell you how long it has been since that file was opened. If it's been more than a few years and you can tell it's something you can live without, get rid of it.

Many people have a sentimental attachment to specific files, especially pictures or media files. If this is the case, you can try curating your work in the form of digital "scrapbooks" that allow you to choose the most important files and delete the rest. First, create subdirectories with a specific name and theme and then move the files you decide to keep into the subdirectory that fits best. Doesn't having a series of virtual scrapbooks make more sense than the clutter you have now?

The Case for Digital Minimalism

In recent years there has been a lot of attention to the *minimalist lifestyle*. While we may not be hoarders as such, virtually everyone has possessions that they don't really need but still have trouble discarding. Do you keep the boxes that new appliances or other purchases come in because you "might need them someday", or do you hang on to old clothes, etc., for sentimental reasons?

For that matter, are you generally more focused on accumulating more possessions in need to impress people or because you think these are things you "should" have to keep up with the latest styles?

People who embrace minimalism insist that their lives become much simpler since they believe that acquiring new experiences is more important than having more stuff in their homes. This way of thinking also means less stress, more time saved from cleaning and home maintenance, and more time with family.

Still, embracing a minimalist lifestyle for the first time can be stressful since it means getting rid of most possessions and learning to live a simpler life, which brings us to *digital minimalism* and the quest to simplify your digital usage as much as possible.

In previous chapters, we have already looked at problems such as digital overwhelm, social media addiction, and digital distractions. We will investigate how to deal with these issues later in the book. But, for now, we will explore ways of getting digital clutter under control and how to cope with digital hoarding if it becomes a problem.

Here are some tips that can help you handle the junk that quickly accumulates for all digital users:

> 1. Don't put off the decluttering process until tomorrow, when you can get started today. Yes, thousands of files need to be examined to see if they are safe to delete. Far too many people decide that digital clutter isn't a problem or think it is too much work to deal with. The sooner you get started, the sooner you will finish.
> 2. Get rid of unused apps and software. Software bloat is a significant problem for users and will likely worsen as

software vendors continue releasing new versions of their products. Not only are they invariably larger, but many companies also bundle in samples of other products they hope you will buy. Think of this as the cyber equivalent of advertising sheets tucked into magazines, etc. Not only does this software bloat often slow down computers, but they consume valuable memory. Most operating systems have uninstall commands allowing for obsolete applications to be removed, but "orphan" files can still be left behind.

3. Organize your Desktop and Documents folders. These can fill up very quickly, especially if you're in the habit of using the Desktop or Documents folders as "scratchpads" to store files pending a cleanup that never happens. Get rid of those unsightly icons and try placing them in special folders you have designated for them. And don't forget to give those folders names that tell you what their purpose is. Don't forget to do the same with your smartphone or tablet since mystery files will bog down your system and keep you from accessing applications faster. There is also less time wasted searching for the files that you need.

4. Make a backup of your most important files. Yes, making more files sounds like a strange way to fight digital clutter, but there is always the chance of deleting something important. Make sure you know what you need to keep and what can be thrown away. You can also store your most important files in the cloud, though you will need an internet connection to access them.

5. Check your email and declutter your inboxes every day. Email inboxes have a way of filling up fast, especially with work email. While you're at it, unsubscribe from email newsletters or other sources of unwanted email that often clog up your inbox daily. And don't hesitate to mark unwanted emails as spam, even if they happen to be from "helpful" sources hoping

to keep you informed about something or another. If you find this a difficult decision to make, just think about all the time it will save you in the future!

6. Get into the digital decluttering habit. Decluttering isn't a one-time chore since new files will pop up before you know it. Whether it's on a monthly or bi-monthly basis, clearing your system of unnecessary files will ensure that your digital life will be much happier and less stressful. If you are part of a work team, try organizing a "spring cleaning" day occasionally so that everyone you work with can eliminate clutter as well.

Remember that the files you delete are still the tip of the iceberg for digital clutter. Now and then, take a good look at your spam folder to get an idea of how much spam you're being deluged with on a regular basis. Digital clutter is just part of the digital overwhelm that affects us all. Regularly decluttering your computer is one way that you can fight back.

In this chapter, we have gone over digital hoarding, digital clutter, and how allowing files to accumulate over time can significantly impact your life. Not only does this mean dealing with the stress of trying to track down old files and making sense of the megabytes of data on your system, but it generally makes users feel more overwhelmed than ever. Therefore, regular decluttering is sensible and one of the most valuable mental health strategies for fighting digital overwhelm.

Chapter Seven

Dealing with Mental Load

In the 1930s, psychologist John Ridley Stroop came up with a rather fiendish research study looking at how visual distractions can get in the way of even simple tasks (Stroop, 1935). In the first part of the study, he asked seventy college undergraduates to read two sheets containing a list of color names, e.g., "Red", "Blue", "Green", "Yellow", etc. The first sheet was printed in black ink, while the second sheet was printed in different colors. Despite the color changes, everyone completed the task without problems.

On the next part of the study, though, Stroop asked a larger pool of subjects to read the sheets as before, along with a third sheet showing a line of squares printed in different ink colors. This time, he asked the subjects to name the color of the ink in which the color names were written. So, for example, the word "red" might have been printed in green ink, and they were expected to answer "green" instead of red.

Stroop found that his subjects took much longer to identify the color of the ink because what they were seeing *conflicted* with the color name they were supposed to supply. They were also much more likely to make mistakes, i.e., reading the word instead of naming the color. However, other experiments showed that this problem only occurred with color names and that subjects had no trouble naming the color of the ink in the squares or if the words were more neutral, i.e., non-color words.

To explain what appeared to be happening, Stroop and later researchers argued that his research subjects only experienced problems when dealing with two separate mental processes that interfered with one another because they were essentially competing for their limited attention spans. As we have already explored in the chapters on multitasking and digital distractions, working memory is extremely limited because of the amount of information we can process at any specific time. Though we can work fine if our brains are focused on a single task, being preoccupied with other things can get in the way of our focus, no matter how minor they may be.

Much like the Stroop effect indicates, we tend not to be very good at shutting out unwanted sensory information. This is particularly true when it interferes with a primary task, which brings us to more recent research dealing with *mental load*.

Though the term has changed meaning over the past few decades, mental load today is usually defined as the impact mental distractors can have on our ability to process data over a given day. These distractors can range from relatively minor sources of stress to whatever significant challenges you might happen to be facing at any given time. Any of these distractors can have an impact on your mental load and your ability to process information at work, home, or anywhere else.

What are the different demands on your time during the average day? This doesn't just mean your daily schedule at work or school (which can be demanding enough in their own way), but also the countless different chores that need to be ticked off on your mental "To Do" list.

Research studies have demonstrated that we spend a large portion of our daily lives thinking about things that are completely unrelated to our immediate environment. These internally aimed thoughts can be goal-directed, meant to pursue a specific purpose, or spontaneous, i.e., "mind wandering." Goal-directed thoughts can involve deliberate planning, creative imagining, or engaging in some form of problem-solving. On the other hand, spontaneous thoughts often arise out of a sense of boredom or wanting to escape from a current reality that you see as unpleasant (think of James Thurber's story about the hapless Walter Mitty and his non-stop daydreaming).

Whatever the reason for these inner thoughts, they often distract people from engaging in tasks they should be focusing on but aren't. As we have already seen in the chapter looking at distracted driving, our overall attention span is limited. Even momentary distractions can be enough to cause problems at work or school. This is another form of mental load, and like any other distractor, can undermine our ability to carry out different tasks.

For working mothers, the term "mental load" has gained new life due to a popular comic strip by the French cartoonist Emma. Her comic, "You Should Have Asked", has virtually become required reading in feminist circles as it details the story of an overworked mom trying to tend to her child at a dinner party as her husband and guests look on. As she tries to handle everything herself, including cooking dinner, it all gets out of hand, and the dinner she is cooking is ruined as a result. When her husband comments on the mess and asks her what she did wrong, the wife eventually explodes at him as he did nothing to help. As the husband then comments that he would have helped if she had asked, the comic then explains that husbands shouldn't have to be *asked* to step up and take responsibility and that moms shouldn't be solely responsible for directing them and planning everything.

As Emma points out in the comic, "when a man expects his partner to ask him to do things, he's viewing her as the manager of household chores" and that he is somehow her underling who needs to be told to do things. As a result, women are often forced to assume an unfair burden of household chores and parenting, in addition to the full-time job they also have. This extra work, and the mental burden that comes with it, is an additional mental load often unique to working parents. This is particularly the case for mothers, who may find themselves worrying about all the different things they need to do in addition to the work tasks that keep them busy during the workday.

Do you need to take your child to the doctor or meet their teacher for some problem or other? Do you have to go shopping for groceries after work? Plan a meal? Pick up a prescription? Call your mother/child/significant other before, during, or after work? Are you feeling too distracted by that argument you had with a family member the night before or some social gathering being planned for the weekend? And what happens when worrying about the different tasks on your mental To-Do list gets in the way of the work you are trying to do?

Much of the psychological toll this kind of mental load can take stems from being unable to 'switch off' or relax. Not only does this prevent you from enjoying leisure time all that much, but it is also often invisible to the people who aren't experiencing it. In addition, this kind of burden can often lead to problems at home, especially if it can be linked to a failure to share responsibilities, which can aggravate emotional tension.

As you might expect, the emotional pressure of these different distractions can profoundly affect your ability to carry out essential tasks. Research has shown that chronic worry can increase the mental load by tying up those inner resources needed for carrying out tasks. In other chapters, we have discussed how limited our working memory can be. We have also seen that competing concerns can reduce mental efficiency due to interfering with everyday tasks. Being preoccupied with emotional problems can have the same impact, leading to a sharp drop in regular cognitive functioning.

Depression and anxiety can be incredibly draining for people trying to function at work, school, or home. Along with the emotions themselves, we can also be preoccupied with the negative thoughts that come with them. These thoughts might involve worrying about things that have happened or things that *might* happen in the future.

Again, allowing mental preoccupations and emotions to increase the mental load people must cope with can have significant consequences for work efficiency and overall health. Though we can reduce this strain by taking frequent breaks and balancing work and home concerns, there are limits to what many employers will allow. This is especially true in jobs requiring people to make endless decisions. We will get into decision fatigue in the next section.

What Is Decision Fatigue?

The mental load can also be a significant source of decision fatigue. The more decisions you make, the harder each new decision becomes. Considering that, the average American adult is estimated to make around 35,000 decisions each day (Sollisch, 2016). Granted, most of these decisions will be trivial ones (e.g., soy vs latte, drive or take the bus to work, etc.). Still, the emotional pressure produced by too much decision-making can have a marked impact on mental and physical health. Some entrepreneurs have taken this knowledge to heart and gone to the extreme of purchasing multiple sets of the same clothes, with the aim to wear the same outfit every day, to cut down on the number of trivial decisions needed to be made every morning and save their brainpower for more important decisions.

According to the Strength Model of Mental Control (Baumeister et al., 1998), every time you decide, you will end up depleting your inner resources, at least to some extent. Much like muscle fatigue after you exert yourself physically, making too many decisions without giving yourself the chance to recover leaves you feeling exhausted, often to the point of questioning every new decision you make. This is decision fatigue in action.

Other factors that can increase the risk of decision fatigue can include the time of day, with studies showing health professionals performing best in the mornings and with their ability to diagnose disease becoming steadily worse over the course of the day. In addition, even something as simple as blood glucose levels can affect decision-making, with decision-making by judges during parole hearings varying widely before or after their mid-day lunch period. Not surprisingly, loss of sleep and physical fatigue can have the same result.

People in professions where their decision-making can have serious consequences, including healthcare workers, air traffic controllers, military personnel, etc., are especially prone to decision fatigue and the problems that can come with it. While there has been surprisingly little research into decision fatigue before this past decade, a recent metanalysis (Pignatiello et al., 2020) has identified the followed characteristics:

Behavioral aspects: Individuals experiencing decision fatigue are more prone to procrastination behaviors, i.e., trying to delay having to decide for as long as possible. They can also become much more passive over time, even to the point of refusing to act to avoid making further decisions. On the other hand, people experiencing decision fatigue can also become much more impulsive and aggressive. Due to the emotional drain that repeated decisions could have on these people, they can display many of the features of what we usually call "burnout".

Cognitive aspects: Decision fatigue can also have a marked impact on mental functioning, including reduced attention span, memory lapses, and sharply reduced problem-solving ability. In other words, the mental load caused by decision fatigue can interfere with normal functioning. As a result, many people affected by decision fatigue are more prone to take mental shortcuts, e.g., choosing the option that seems most effortless rather than making the best possible choice.

Physiological attributes: Similar to other forms of chronic stress, decision fatigue can drain physical and mental endurance. For example, a series of laboratory studies examined the effects of decision-making on physical endurance by asking research participants to make a series of choices about shopping for consumer goods or college courses. Then they compared them with a control group on a *cold pressor test* (evaluates the length of time an individual can withstand the discomfort of having their hand submerged in ice-water). The researchers found that the decision-making group had less overall endurance than the control group, indicating how decision fatigue can drain inner resources (Vohs et al., 2008).

How to Deal with Decision Fatigue

While more hospital emergency departments take decision fatigue seriously, there are still limits to how many breaks nurses and doctors can receive each day. This was especially true in areas hard hit by the COVID-19 pandemic, with medical staff facing extreme pressures to make multiple medical decisions each day. This pressure significantly impacted personnel, many of whom risk burnout regularly.

In a 2020 review, Moorehouse (2020) proposed a series of tips for reducing decision fatigue. While specifically aimed at health professionals, the same tips can be applied for anyone having to make too many decisions:

1. Don't be afraid to delegate tasks to other people, whether a work team member or a spouse who isn't doing enough to handle daily responsibilities. You don't have to do it all yourself.
2. Establish regular routines and guidelines to narrow down the choices you must make. Reducing these choices to one or two options can reduce the stress a bit.
3. Don't be afraid to discuss your possible choices with other people and get their feedback on what you should do. If you are a student, this can be a parent or teacher. For working mothers, this can be a spouse or friend.
4. If necessary, put off the decision you must make to another day. That way, at least you can come back to it with fresh eyes. Don't confuse this with procrastinating, however. If a decision must be made, then make it as soon as you realistically can.
5. Recognize that some tasks can wait until you have thought over the options a little more. Don't be afraid to leave a task undone for a while to give your brain some time to percolate

over the different possibilities. It might make deciding a little easier later.

6. Reduce the overall number of decisions you need to make each day. Along with delegating many of these decisions, you can also plan ahead. That can include preparing your wardrobe and meals in advance to reduce your mental load a bit. Use a day planner to schedule appointments, responsibilities, etc., so you aren't frantically trying to keep track of everything you are supposed to be doing. An online resource such as Google Calendar can be invaluable and can be synced with all your digital devices as needed.

7. Take breaks! Break up your day into manageable chunks with some time spent away from your desk and your computer. Don't be afraid to mute your phone either, at least while you're sitting somewhere drinking coffee.

Can Digital Devices Help with Mental Load?

Over the past two decades, we have seen a massive rise in digital technology and watched it transform virtually all aspects of life. But how effective is it in helping people of all ages cope with the enormous influx of new data that this digital revolution is making possible? Digital competence, or digital literacy, has been widely studied in recent years, especially in terms of lifetime learning. It appears to play a vital role in allowing people to cope with the mental load. The European Union has already identified digital competence as being just as much a fundamental skill as reading and writing.

Not only is digital competence crucial for students hoping to succeed in higher education. Virtually all white-collar jobs and a rising number of blue-collar jobs also depend on digital technology for processing and creating information, not to mention passing that information on to others. This has led to a massive influx of new time-saving and labor-saving apps to make life easier, both at work and home. It has also spawned a new industry as more and more new apps become available on smartphones, tablets, laptops, and even digital watches. For that matter, we are also seeing a rise in new apps for use in cars and other devices as the Internet of Things truly takes off.

Many of these new apps are specifically tailored to improve users' mental health. This includes meditation and mindfulness training, scheduling, keeping track of social contacts, or generally staying in control of life, which seem to be getting more complicated from one day to the next.

This chapter has reviewed different aspects of mental and cognitive load and how they affect mental and physical health. This has included looking at early research and how competing mental tasks can interfere with one another, given our limited working memory and problem-solving capacity. More recent studies examine the impact of mental interference experienced by working mothers and others dealing with multiple demands on time and energy that can impact their ability to engage in regular work functioning. This chapter also addressed other forms of mental load, including the effects of worry and decision fatigue and how they compromise mental and physical health and our ability to focus on mental activities at work, school, and home. Finally, we looked at how digital competence can provide a way of coping with mental load through greater use of online and digital apps for simplifying many aspects of our daily lives.

Chapter Eight

Coping with Isolation

At the age of fifteen, a Japanese adolescent identified in a 2006 New York Times news story only as Takeshi withdrew into his bedroom and, for much of the next four years of his life, refused to leave except for going to the bathroom. Spending 23 hours a day in his tiny bedroom eating food prepared by his mother, Takeshi refused to attend school or get a job. Instead, he devoted himself to watching television and listening to music by Radiohead and Nirvana. As he would later admit in that same media interview, his music choices were shaped by his somber mood. "Anything that was dark and sounded desperate," he said. Finally, Takeshi eventually decided to leave his bedroom and rejoin the world. He even enrolled in a job-training program and largely credited his taste in music for return to society. "Don't laugh, but musicians really helped me, especially Radiohead," he said through an interpreter. "That's what encouraged me to leave my room."

In Japan, this phenomenon is known as hikikomori which means "pulling inward" or "being confined", and cases like Takeshi's are far more common than you might think. Along with being a part of Japanese culture (with other occurrences being reported in countries such as South Korea, Taiwan, and Brazil), many adolescents and young adults under the age of twenty-one have deliberately chosen to withdraw entirely from the world with little outside contact but their parents.

That doesn't appear to apply to online communication, and online meeting sites are becoming increasingly popular. One such site, Hikikomori Platform, was founded in 2019. According to its founder, Takahiro Tajima, there has been a sharp rise in online meetings since it allows shut-ins to interact with other hikikomori and help them prepare to rejoin society.

While the actual incidence of hikikomori is still hard to estimate since not all cases come to the attention of government agencies, there seems little doubt that such cases have soared in the past two decades. According to some sources suggesting that there may be millions in Japan, this number is controversial given the lack of a clear definition. The number of hikikomori cases reported may include older adults who have voluntarily withdrawn from the world or suffer from a broader mental disorder that can mimic the symptoms.

However common it is in Japan, hikikomori seems to have become a part of Japan's popular culture along with otaku, which is the Japanese equivalent of "geek" or "nerd". Both terms have been heavily associated with Japanese manga culture. They are often linked together in the media to describe young people so obsessed with manga that they completely shut out the world. Other derogatory terms often linked to the hikikomori phenomenon are *freeter* or *furita* (equivalent to "slackers" in Western countries) and *parasaito shinguru* or parasite singles who live off their parents to avoid facing adult responsibilities. Whatever the term used, the stigma surrounding *hikikomori* is severe enough to reinforce the social anxiety driving young people to shut out the world and often preventing parents from seeking help for their children. And parents themselves are often blamed for "enabling" their children's behavior.

While hikikomori is primarily considered a Japan-only problem, that seems to be changing in recent years. It is likely a sign of the time that the venerable Oxford English Dictionary added a new entry for hikikomori in 2010. In addition, international surveys of psychiatrists in Australia, the United States, France, Spain, Italy, and Brazil have already identified hikikomori cases in all those countries (Kato et al., 2019). Granted, the most extreme occurrences appear to be linked with other mental health issues such as depression, social anxiety, and schizophrenia. However, the kind of pathological social withdrawal seen in hikikomori cases seems to be occurring in many countries worldwide.

So, why does hikikomori appear to be spreading around the world? In a recent analysis of the global hikikomori phenomenon (Kato et al., 2019), clinical researchers suggest that the rise of the Internet and the impact that modern digital technology has on how young people interact with the world may be a factor.

Not only does online gaming allow children and adolescents to do all their gaming virtually. There also seems to be an overall shift away from "direct" ways of interacting with the world (i.e., going out and socializing) towards more "indirect" interaction using digital sources. Now, actual face-to-face social contact is becoming less important due to social media, email, texting, TikTok videos, etc.

On the other hand, young people are now being exposed to forms of bullying and harassment over which they have even less control than real-life bullying. Not only can they be subjected to cyberbullying and cyberstalking by people they have never met. The often-vicious abuse they receive can severely undermine mental health and make victims even less likely to seek help as a result.

One of the things that makes hikikomori and other forms of social withdrawal so hard to overcome is that the longer young people remain isolated, the harder it is to reintegrate into regular social life. Though treatment programs to help hikikomori youth are common in Japan, it is still primarily a hidden epidemic in other countries, and finding specialized help will be considerably more challenging as a result.

While this extreme social isolation is still relatively rare (so far), social isolation is becoming more common, primarily due to the availability of digital devices taking the "social" out of social interaction. We will explore some of the possible reasons for this later in this chapter.

Is Digital Addiction Making Us More Isolated?

Though we have already explored the Internet and digital addiction in earlier chapters, we still need to understand what addiction is and how it can shape the way people live their lives. According to the American Society of Addiction Medicine, addiction is a primary disruption of mood, behavior, and functioning, and along with compulsive cravings, can lead to negative life impacts in the major spheres of living.

While we usually think of this in terms of drug or alcohol addiction, it is also possible to become psychologically dependent on pleasurable activities such as gambling or overeating. There is still some controversy over whether addiction to behaviors can affect the brain similarly to substance use. Still, research suggests that repetitive behaviors can influence the brain's reward structures based in the mesolimbic and prefrontal cortexes in much the same way that they respond to physically addictive substances.

These same complex brain structures do appear to be linked to digital addiction. Though digital addiction can take different forms, including protracted Internet, smartphone, or video game use, being glued to a screen does appear to create a reward pattern like what people experience at slot machines. Like gambling with the possibility of winning, the prospect of enjoyable social media posts, texts, or content can boost dopamine levels to produce a sensation of euphoria. This sensation, in turn, reinforces the need to stay online.

In many ways, the Internet itself can be seen as the world's most giant slot machine since it operates on what is basically a variable reinforcement schedule that increases the likelihood of long-term dependence. Since you never know what you are going to find on the Internet or how pleasurable or unpleasurable the content will be, the unpredictable nature of Web surfing keeps our brains tuned to an elevated state of stimulation along with our dopamine and cortisol levels.

And, because the prospect of reward is so unpredictable, digital use is tough to fade over time, a process known as "extinction" if you recall your introductory Psychology class. Since we can expect to find something pleasurable on the Internet sooner or later, we are basically rewarded- a principle long recognized by internet advertisers, bloggers, YouTube, and TikTok video producers, etc.

The smartphone is an exceptionally addictive digital device since it has already become the primary internet access portal for over half the world's population. Not only do smartphones allow instant access to friends, relatives, and strangers, but the constant notifications we receive via smartphone help reinforce the sense of FOMO that keeps us online much of the day.

internet addiction, much like gambling or compulsive eating, is reinforced by the *reward deficiency syndrome* that makes everyday life seem much blander and less exciting than what we experience when engaged in these pleasurable activities. In a real sense, the longer we spend online, the less satisfying other activities such as face-to-face socializing, work, and school become by comparison. And the more compulsive internet use becomes, the less time and attention we spend on regular activities.

Prolonged internet use also creates an interesting paradox since it allows us to become connected to larger internet communities while cutting us off from our regular family and friendship networks. While this sounds much like the hikikomori described earlier in this chapter, most people dealing with internet addiction rarely go this far unless they are dealing with other mental health problems such as severe depression or social anxiety.

What Is The Digital Dozen?

In a recent overview on digital addiction, psychologist David Greenfield (2021) identified what he called the "Digital Dozen," a list of twelve factors that make smartphones and other digital devices so addictive:

Accessibility – There is never an "off period" for the Internet. No matter when you want to access it, day or night, seven days a week, the Internet will always be there.

Intensity and stimulation (content addiction) – The Internet is filled with stimulating and intoxicating content, readily available to (virtually) anyone who wants it. Granted, many sites pay at least some lip service to restrict content to people over eighteen and otherwise considered to be adults, but finding content parents might deem inappropriate for children is rarely a challenge. For those seeking content considered immoral or illegal in many places, there is also the Dark net that places few restrictions on such shocking content.

Novel and dynamic content – The Internet constantly changes with new and appealing content coming online. Not only does this reinforce the FOMO that drives people to spend as much time online as they can.

Dissociation – It is very easy to lose track of time when you are engaged in something that absorbs all your attention. If you have ever been inside a casino, you will notice the total absence of clocks or windows that might provide gamblers with cues concerning how much time is passing. Though internet providers don't have this option, it is still to their advantage to make their content as absorbing as possible to encourage people to stay online longer.

Allowing people to connect – Smartphones, social media, and bulletin boards allow users to stay in contact with friends, family, and acquaintances and even allow them to form new online friendships with people that they might have never met otherwise. Still, this online contact doesn't provide the same "nutritional" value that face-to-face contact does, even if it seems enough for many users.

Perceived anonymity – One of the greatest draws that the Internet provides is the opportunity to hide your identity. Still, there is much less anonymity on the Internet than most people believe. Many internet service providers and sites routinely compile enormous amounts of data that can be sold to any customer.

Disinhibition – Along with this greater sense of anonymity is the sense of freedom that can come with it. This anonymity often allows people to "reinvent themselves" in ways they would have been otherwise afraid to do. Though this seems harmless enough on the surface, we see an epidemic of racist, sexist, and homophobic abuse coming from many people who would never dream of being so open in real life.

The story that has no end – Information on the Internet has no boundaries. Since our brains need to resolve incomplete stories, we rely on hyperlinks, and there is always a new one to click. This need led us to keep clicking to find out more, which content providers rely on to keep us hooked.

Cost – Though digital devices and internet services cost money, spending time on the Internet is cheap once that initial payment is made. Even in developing nations, people living in poverty typically rely on smartphones for business, social, and entertainment purposes.

Instant gratification – The faster we get reinforced and rewarded by a substance or behavior, the quicker we become addicted. This means that the shorter the time between clicking on a link or getting a response from a digital app, the more addictive it becomes.

Interactivity – Every interaction we have on the Internet, every search, and every time we use an app, appears to be under our control. While the Internet's reward structure shapes our behavior, the sense of control that we have over our digital devices keeps us from realizing that.

Variable ratio reinforcement schedule – As we have already seen earlier in this chapter, the "maybe" factor reinforces the need to stay online. While not every interaction will be rewarding, the anticipation of eventually being rewarded makes it more challenging to eliminate the need to keep us coming back for more.

Why the Smartphone Makes us Addicts

Though digital devices and the Internet have evolved dramatically over the past ten years alone, the smartphone has become the single most significant game-changer. By 2019 alone, an estimated eighty-one percent of all Americans owned a smartphone. The Internet has now become almost completely untethered from the bulky machines, complicated cables, and slow dial-up that marked its humble beginnings. Though internet cafes can still be found virtually anywhere you go globally, there are few, if any, services they offer that can't be replicated with a smartphone you can carry with you anywhere.

When looking over the "digital dozen" listed above, it's easy to see that the smartphone is likely the single most addictive digital device of all. Getting a phone notification, whether it's a ping, a buzz, a pre-set ringtone, or feeling it vibrate, can instantly signal that we need to drop everything and answer to see what new content we are being offered. Much like the bells and flashing lights of a slot machine, this learned behavior is incredibly difficult to resist, even if you happen to be in a classroom, work meeting, driving, etc., which is likely more important. Knowing anything about Ivan Pavlov's work with dogs being conditioned to salivate at the sound of a bell, you will probably relate this to how often you check your phone over the course of the day.

Whenever you hear the ping of an upcoming text message, a ring tone, a social media update, or an email, that small hit of dopamine it generates well ensures that you will be distracted from whatever else you are doing as well. Even if you are driving with a hands-free Bluetooth connection allowing you to answer a call, dividing your attention means reducing your focus on the road, even temporarily. The same applies if you are engaged in anything else worthwhile, and you find yourself becoming more isolated as a result. And that isolation can become a habit over time.

Though there is still an active debate over the exact nature of the Internet or digital addiction and its definition, treatment programs can be found worldwide. For example, in South Korea, China, and Taiwan, the estimated prevalence of internet addiction among adolescents ranges from 1.6 to 11.3 percent. Similar numbers are reported in the United States (Greenfield, 2021), and treatment services are in high demand.

How Isolated Are We Becoming Because of Digital Devices?

Though we have already discussed Dr. Jean Twenge's research into the rise of overall unhappiness among young people since 2012, much of her research also shows how isolated the "iGen generation" is becoming. A recent study (Twenge et al., 2019), used representative samples of U.S. adolescents aged thirteen to eighteen and compared samples of teenagers entering college in 1976 and 2017.

They found that iGen adolescents in the 2010s spent far less time on face-to-face interactions with people their own age than any of the previous generations surveyed. These interactions included rudimentary social interactions like getting together, attending parties, dating, visiting movies, etc. College-bound high school seniors in 2016 also reported spending an hour less a day socializing than their 1976 counterparts.

Adolescents also showed a sharp rise in reported loneliness from 2011 onward compared to previous years. As you might expect, adolescents reporting high social media use and low in-person social interaction were most likely to disclose the most loneliness.

But loneliness can strike at any age. According to a 2018 survey commissioned by Cigna Insurance (Cigna, 2018), nearly half of the 20,000 Americans surveyed reported frequent loneliness, with Generation Z adults (18-22) showing the highest loneliness scores. While social media use was not considered a cause of loneliness, Generation Z adults were also much more likely to be heavy users of social media and less likely to report having good physical and mental health.

Adolescents and young adults are especially prone to developing mental health issues due to the importance of social relationships during this critical period of emotional development. The iGen generation seems more connected socially and "plugged in" to digital content via social media, online gaming, and internet use than any previous generation. However, the increased loneliness they are experiencing suggests online relationships are not meaningful enough to stave off loneliness.

This information appears to fit well with the interpersonal-connection-behaviors framework proposed by Jenna Clark and her colleagues (Clark et al., 2017). According to this framework, online social network sites can be beneficial to make *meaningful* social connections, such as forming genuine online friendships or remaining in contact with friends and family members from real life. This type of use typically works best for people who already have good social networks and use the Internet to reinforce those networks.

For people who already feel isolated and lack strong social networks, using the Internet to compensate for this sense of isolation usually has the opposite effect. Not only are these people prone to "Facebook depression" due to their need to compare themselves to other people online (who are typically seen as having happier and more successful lives), but they are also prone to "social snacking." This term essentially means lurking on other strangers' profiles, enjoying the pictures and videos of their children or pets, congratulating them for positive developments, and generally getting the temporary benefit that comes of it, but still end up feeling lonelier than ever.

Research suggests a strong link between social media use and loneliness, even in adults. However, this link works both ways; not only are lonely people more likely to turn to social media to form social connections, but the time spent on social media can also increase loneliness.

Though it is certainly possible to become part of different online communities and have hundreds, if not thousands, of followers, there is an apparent trade-off between the number of potential relationships online and the actual *quality* of those relationships. While most research studies looking into loneliness in adults have focused on seniors, chronic loneliness, whether it is aggravated by internet use or not, can have severe effects on mental and physical health.

Cyberbullying, Online Abuse, and the Fight for Self-Esteem

When exploring the link between internet use and loneliness, we also need to consider how easily it can be used for anonymous attacks on vulnerable users. While there is nothing new about bullying, especially among young people trying to form social relationships as a part of growing up, the rise of digital media over the past two decades has been accompanied by the appearance of cyberbullying as a significant social problem.

Online harassment is prevalent for women and members of sexual or racial minority groups, given that many harassers take advantage of anonymity to engage in extremist language and threats. Harmful bullying behaviors can include posting rumors, making crude sexual remarks, hate speech, or releasing personal information, as well as revealing images aimed at humiliating victims.

Despite the severe consequences of cyberbullying, including many high-profile suicides in recent years, local police departments are typically ill-equipped to track down perpetrators. Also, since laws against cyberbullying often vary across different jurisdictions, actual prosecution is rare.

While at least half of all young people have experienced cyberbullying in some form, the ones who spend the most time online are particularly vulnerable. Though most social media platforms, including Facebook and Twitter, have policies in place to discourage online abuse, the ease with which cyberbullies can switch to new anonymous accounts means that such attacks are rarely stopped for long.

For young people who already feel isolated, the psychological consequences of cyberbullying can be severe. Not only do victims develop a lower sense of self-esteem, but they can also become depressed and suicidal if they are unable to fight back against anonymous harassment. As a result, they often become even more isolated and avoid family and friends who might help them cope. Though an estimated twenty to forty percent of adolescents are believed to be victims of cyberbullying worldwide, the actual number will likely never be known since many victims hide their abuse.

Adolescent victims of cyberbullying typically show changes in their eating and sleeping patterns and become more isolated in general. This isolation also increases the risk of suicide, especially if the victim does not feel that anyone can help them.

While cyberbullying will almost certainly become more of a problem in the future as young people become more dependent on their digital devices, we seem no closer to finding real solutions to the damage it can do. Only time will tell what the future will bring.

How To Cope with Digital Isolation

While there is no single solution for the increase in loneliness and isolation that seems to have developed in the past decade, recent research (Cigna, 2018) has identified the following lifestyle tips for improving physical and mental health:

> 1. Strike a good balance between digital and face-to-face social interactions. That means getting out more and finding in-person activities that can satisfy the FOMO people of all ages experience. This may be a challenge for naturally shy people or people dealing with social anxiety. Still, those who have daily meaningful in-person interactions report being far less lonely than those whose main interactions are online.
> 2. Develop a regular exercise routine. Along with feelings of loneliness, people who spend much of their time online are also prone to physical problems resulting from not getting enough exercise. Going to a gym regularly can also be a source of social interaction, especially if you participate in structured training with others. Check out the different exercise classes available at your local gym or community center. It is also essential to see your doctor regularly and get medical advice before starting any exercise program.
> 3. Develop a regular sleep schedule. People who feel isolated often neglect sleep or spend too much time sleeping at odd hours. Additionally, as we already saw in a previous chapter, spending too much time watching a digital screen at odd hours can disrupt your sleep schedule by affecting melatonin levels in

the brain. Try to avoid screens entirely during the hours when you are supposed to be sleeping.

4. Take regular digital breaks. Try to limit the amount of time you spend online by scheduling regular rest breaks after every hour or so. These breaks mean getting away from online matters as much as possible, whether by taking a walk outside or doing some other real-world activity to take yourself out of that digital headspace and remind yourself that the real world still exists. Even in the workplace, it is still possible to find non-digital things to do that take you away from your desk. That includes exercise breaks and going to the gym on your lunch hour if possible. Even a quick walk around the block to get some fresh air can help relieve digital stress.

5. Be more social in general – Spend time talking with friends, family, and coworkers. Try to engage them in the kind of conversations you might have online, and you might find the intimacy you are often missing as a result.

6. Don't be afraid to ask for help – For many people, dealing with digital isolation may be too difficult to solve on their own. Issues such as severe social anxiety or painful shyness may require professional help to overcome. If you're still in school, don't be afraid to talk to a guidance counselor or school nurse about what is happening. Your family doctor may also be able to refer you to someone in the area who can help. Additionally, there are websites for organizations offering help for people of all ages to cope with emotional issues.

This chapter has explored why isolation seems to have grown more common than ever over the past decade. The hikikomori phenomenon, which once was unique to Japan, now appears to spread worldwide. We see social isolation become an increasing problem for people of all ages as they become more dependent on digital media and see their real-world connections slowly shrink along the way. This trend is especially true for adolescents and young adults who have become dependent on the Internet for much of their social functioning. Whether this is a case of lonely people turning to the Internet for social interactions or people who become lonelier due to online social contacts crowding out face-to-face contact with friends and family, the result appears to be the same. This chapter also explored the issue of digital addiction and how the variable reinforcement provided by online content can have the same impact on brain chemistry due to the psychological dependence that results. We also explored cyberbullying and other forms of online harassment and how they can lead to severe psychological issues which can reinforce loneliness. Finally, we went into some of the different ways of fighting digital isolation and striking a proper balance between online and in-person socializing as well as learning to be healthier and happier as a result.

Conclusion

After a public charter school in California experienced its first-ever cyberbullying incident, a parent of one of the children at the school, Diana Garber, offered to help. As a recent M.A. in Media Psychology and Social Change, Garber joined with the school principal, Shaheer Faltas, to launch a new kind of digital literacy program for the students at the school. Based on the weekly Civics classes already being held, Garber and Faltas established the first "Cyber Civics" class with input from academics and educators around the country. Along with teaching ethical and critical thinking, Cyber Civics also teaches children about media literacy and information literacy, as well as helping children to make sense of a digital world. Students are also taught about the dark side of the Internet, including coping with cyberbullying, hate speech, and privacy violations. The course also includes take-home projects for students to carry out with their families.

Given its popularity, Cyber Civics is now being taught to thousands of children worldwide. Diana Garber also published a book in 2019 titled "Raising Humans in a Digital World: Helping Kids Build a Healthy Relationship with Technology" and plays an active role in the Cyber Civics movement. She has also established a new website Cyberwise.org in 2011, as a companion site to

Cyber Civics. Visitors can learn more about Cyber Civics, find online resources to teach good digital citizenship to children, and download a parent-oriented version of the Cyber Wise curriculum to use with their children.

However, Cyber Civics is hardly unique in warning about the potential risks of cyber technology to children and adolescents. If anything, the need to deal with digital overwhelm has spawned a new industry in recent years. Along with internet addiction treatment centers springing up worldwide, there are also programs such as Cyber Wise and a growing number of books on the need for digital health. There are even vacation resorts whose main appeal is the ability to escape from digital devices, at least for a little while.

Throughout this book, we have explored the importance of digital wellness and many of the online risks that can undermine mental and physical health for people of all ages. This includes how the rising dependence that children and adolescents have on digital devices has spawned an iGen generation that seems to be growing steadily more isolated and unhappy despite having access to more information than previous generations had ever dreamed possible.

We also looked at issues such as Facebook depression, cyberbullying, sexting, online hate speech and what that can mean to young people's self-esteem, and the role this can play in later problems such as substance abuse and suicide.

But the digital revolution is not just affecting the iGen generation. Baby Boomers and Generation Xers are also finding their lives being transformed. Nearly all adults now own at least one digital device, and most of them describe themselves as "constant checkers" who see the need to stay on top of their email, social media accounts, and other online sources. They also see this as a source of considerable stress in their lives.

Many of the same issues affecting younger users apply to older adults, especially when dealing with mean-spirited, harassing, or otherwise upsetting content. Unfortunately, for women and sexual minorities, cyber-harassment and cyber-stalking are all too familiar despite efforts by social media sites to rein in abuse.

The recent pandemic and the need for social distancing have made people more dependent on digital devices than ever. There has been a sharp rise in remote working, visual learning, and the use of social media to fill in for the loss of face-to-face social contact that many people were experiencing. This change meant that more people than ever spent much of their daily lives glued to a computer screen with all the problems that could come with it.

One prominent example of how dependent we have become on digital devices is the recent rise in distracted driving accidents. As we have already seen earlier, data from the National Highway Traffic Safety Administration shows that an estimated 78 percent of all crashes and 65 percent of near-crashes in the United States alone were due to distracted driving, particularly distracted driving involving smartphones. While traffic fatalities are decreasing due to better automotive safety features, one in six are believed to be due to drivers using digital devices for phone calls, texting, email, etc.

Along with recognizing the risks posed by digital distractions on the road, digital devices are also linked to a range of mental health issues, many of which have gained their own names, such as "Facebook depression," "technostress," and "digital burnout," to name just a few. These problems are likely to become even worse in the future, given the increasing dependence on digital devices and the prospect of even greater connectiveness with the machines around us as the Internet of Things lives up to its promise.

As we have also seen, one of the main drivers of this rising epidemic of technostress and digital burnout stems from the sense of digital overwhelm as we try to filter out the tremendous volume of information provided by the Internet and social media. In addition, the intense fear of missing out (FOMO) that keeps us online, as well as our own need to stay connected and well-informed about the world around us, means spending even more time online. Not only does this crowd out our regular social contacts with friends and family, but the loss of intimate contact that online content and interactions cannot replace.

To deal with digital overwhelm, we are often driven to take "shortcuts" by attempting to multitask, despite the evidence from cognitive psychology showing that humans are simply not wired that way.

The critical thing to remember about our relationship with digital devices and the Internet is that we are still coming to terms with something incredibly new. While the iGen generation has lived with digital devices all their lives, even those of us who remember a time before the Internet, smartphones, and tablets know there is no going back. It is up to us to establish how we will live with this rapidly changing technology.

Future developments, such as the Internet of Things, are likely to cause even more disruption to our daily lives. However, it is still possible to balance our online and real-world lives in a way that doesn't seriously undermine our mental and physical health. Therefore, it is essential for everyone who relies on the Internet and social media to establish basic ground rules to prevent many complex problems discussed in this book.

Here are some suggestions:

1. Start by setting boundaries for yourself and your children. That means not being afraid to turn off your digital devices and spend more time on real-world activities. Limit yourself to a set number of hours online and stick to that limit. You can try not to check your email or social media after a fixed time each evening. Which time you pick is up to you, but don't be afraid to stick to it, no matter how tempted you are by the pop-up notice or buzz on your smartphone telling you there is a new email.
2. Keep digital devices out of your bedroom. A smartphone in arm's reach may be all right for emergencies, but you don't need a tablet or a flat-screen TV that might disrupt your sleep schedule.
3. Establish at least one "free day" a week to get away from your digital devices. You can live without social media or email for at least twenty-four hours, and if you can't, then accept that your digital dependence is more severe than you thought.
4. Come to terms with FOMO. Yes, exciting things are happening in the digital world but don't get caught up in all the latest memes. Recognize that you must set limits on yourself and that your life won't be any worse for missing out on the latest online fad. And be careful about the memes you're passing around to friends. Not every news story that seems believable is true.
5. Curb your need to stay informed. Also, set limits for yourself and your need to keep up on the latest news. Check the news once a day to keep up on what is happening but otherwise, stop scanning the news sites constantly. If the world is coming to an end, you will likely get plenty of advance notice anyway.
6. Shut off push alerts and control the notifications you get. Most of those notices will be advertisements or unimportant to you anyway. And no matter how attractive they may

seem, don't click on strange ads or download files that seem unfamiliar, especially if you don't know who is sending them.

7. Stay safe online. That means keeping antivirus and antispam software up to date and learning to deal with spam, malware, and all the other traps you might encounter. Not only will this help you avoid a lot of the digital distractions already out there, but it will keep your private data private and save you from risks such as identity theft.

8. Commit to digital detox regularly. Put your phone in airplane mode, leave your tablet at home, and try taking a walk or going to the gym occasionally. The Internet will still be there when you get back.

These are just a few suggestions to get your life back into balance, but in the end, it is up to you to establish those ground rules and stick to them. Don't hesitate to teach these ground rules to your children since they will likely be the ones who need them most.

As a final note, remember what we talked about in the introduction. Though your memories of a pre-digital world are likely fading, we are still in the very early stages of this digital revolution, unlike anything previous generations have been forced to manage. That means that you are probably not prepared for what is coming next. New changes such as the Internet of Things, blockchain, and quantum computing will keep on transforming life as we know it, and it is crucial to be ready to deal with these changes as they happen. Whether or not you want to admit it, you and your children will be living in a digital world for the rest of your lives. How you learn to handle it, and what you teach your children to help them handle it, is up to you.

Thank you for reading!

Thank you for your purchase. If you enjoyed this book, feel free to leave a review on Amazon. This will help us to continue to provide great books, and it will help our potential buyers make confident buying decisions. We will be forever grateful, thank you in advance!

https://www.rpbook.co.uk/azr/B09S FMPB9D

Also by Jessie Fields:

https://getbook.at/Rest

References

Andreassen, C.S. (2015). Online social network site addiction: A comprehensive review. *Current Addiction Reports,* 2 (2) (pp. 175-184). doi:10.1007/s40429-015-0056-9

Anfinsen, J. (2014, April 29). E-hoarding is a new phenomenon that is quickly spreading amongst computer users. *WPTV.* Archived from the original on (2014, Aug 8). Retrieved (2014, April 8). https://web.archive.org/web/20140808141115/http://www.wptv.com/news/science-tech/e-hoarding-is-a-new-phenomenon-spreading-like-a-computer-virus-for-users

Baker, Z. G., Krieger, H., & LeRoy, A. S. (2016). Fear of missing out: Relationships with depression, mindfulness, and physical symptoms. *Translational Issues in Psychological Science,* 2(3), (pp. 275-282). https://doi.org/10.1037/tps0000075

Baumeister, R. F., Bratslavsky, E., Muraven, M., Tice, D. M. (1998). Ego depletion: is the active self a limited resource? *J Pers Soc Psychol* 74(5) (pp. 1252-65). doi:10.1037//0022-3514.74.5.1252

Brod, C. (1984). Technostress: The Human Cost of the Computer Revolution. *Reading, MA: Addison-Wesley.* ISBN-10:0201112116

Cheng, C., Lau, Y., Chan, L., & Luk, J. W. (2021). Prevalence of social media addiction across 32 nations: Meta-analysis with subgroup analysis of classification schemes and cultural values, *Addictive Behaviors, 117*. https://doi.org/10.1016/j.addbeh.2021.106845

Cigna Insurance, (2018). *Cigna U.S. Loneliness Index Survey.* Retrieved from: https://www.cigna.com/static/www-cigna-com/docs/about-us/newsroom/studies-and-reports/combatting-loneliness/loneliness-survey-2018-full-report.pdf

Clark, J. L., Algoe, S. B., & Green, M. C. (2017). Social Network Sites and Well-Being: The Role of Social Connection. *Current Directions in Psychological Science, 27*(1) (pp. 32-37). https://doi.org/10.1177/0963721417730833

Dong, Y., Hu, Z., Uchimura, K., & Murayama, N. (2011). Driver Inattention Monitoring System for Intelligent Vehicles: A Review. *IEEE Transactions on Intelligent Transportation Systems, 12*(2) (pp. 596-614). https://doi.org/10.1109/TITS.2010.2092770

Finley, J. R., Benjamin, A. S., & McCarley, J. S. (2014). Metacognition of multitasking: How well do we predict the costs of divided attention? *Journal of Experimental Psychology: Applied, 20*(2). doi:10.1037/xap0000010

Froese, A. D., Carpenter, C. N., Inman, D. A., Schooley, J. R., Barnes, R. B., Brecht, P. W., & Chacon, J. D. (2012, June). Effects of classroom cell phone use on expected and actual learning. *College Student Journal, 46*(2) (pp. 323-332).

Garber, D. (2019). Raising Humans in a Digital World: Helping Kids Build a Healthy Relationship with Technology. *Amazon.* ISBN-10:0814439799, ISBN-13:978-0814439791

Graham, A., & Sahlberg, P. (2021). Growing Up Digital Australia: Phase 2 technical report. Sydney, Australia: Gonski Institute for Education, UNSW

Greenfield, D. N. (2021). Digital distraction: What makes the internet and smartphone so addictive? In S. M. Lane & P. Atchley (Eds.), *Human capacity in the attention economy* (pp. 27-47). American Psychological Association. https://doi.org/10.1037/0000208-003

Holmes, T. H., & Rahe, R. H., (1967, August). The Social Readjustment Rating Scale. *Journal of Psychosomatic Research, 11*(2) (pp. 213-218) https://doi.org/10.1016/0022-3999(67)90010-4

Hu, E. (2013, October 10). New Numbers Back Up Our Obsession With Phones. *NPR National Public Radio.* Retrieved from https://www.npr.org/sections/alltechconsidered/2013/10/09/230867952/new-numbers-back-up-our-obsession-with-phones

Kato, T. A., Kanba, S., & Teo, A. R., (2019). Hikikomori: Multidimensional understanding, assessment, and future international perspectives. *Psychiatry Clin Neurosci. 73*(8) (pp.427-440). doi:10.1111/pcn.12895

Kushlev, K., & Dunn, E. W., (2015). Checking e-mail less frequently reduces stress. *Computers in Human Behavior, 43* (pp. 220–228). doi:10.1016/j.chb.2014.11.005

Mandel, M. (2005, October 3). The real reasons you're working so hard. *Business Week.* (pp. 60–67).

Monteith, S., Glenn, T., Geddes, J., Severus, E., Whybrow, P. C., & Bauer, M. (2021). Internet of things issues related to psychiatry. *Int J Bipolar Disord, 9*(11). https://doi.org/10.1186/s40345-020-00216-y

Moorehouse, A. (2020). Decision fatigue: less is more when making choices with patients. *The British journal of general practice : the journal of the Royal College of General Practitioners, 70*(697), (pp. 399). https://doi.org/10.3399/bjgp20X711989

Oakes, K. (2019, January 7). Why it pays to declutter your digital life. *BBC Future.* https://www.bbc.com/future/article/20190104-are-you-a-digital-hoarder

Pashler, H. (1994). Dual-task interference in simple tasks: Data and theory. *Psychological Bulletin, 116*(2), (pp. 220–244). doi:10.1037/0033-2909.116.2.220.

Pignatiello, G. A., Martin, R. J., & Hickman, R. L. Jr., (2020). Decision fatigue: A conceptual analysis. *Journal of health psychology, 25*(1), (pp. 123–135). https://doi.org/10.1177/1359105318763510

Prince, K. A. (2018). Digital leadership: transitioning into the digital age. *PhD thesis.* Queensland, Australia: James Cook University. doi:10.25903/5d2bdd672c0e5

The Radicati Group, Inc., (2017). Email Statistics Report, 2017-2021. Retrieved from https://www.radicati.com/wp/wp-content/uploads/2017/01/Email-Statistics-Report-2017-2021-Executive-Summary.pdf

Reed, J., Hirsh-Pasek, K., & Golinkoff, R. M. (2017). Learning on hold: Cell phones sidetrack parent-child interactions. *Developmental Psychology, 53*(8), (pp. 1428-1436). http://dx.doi.org/10.1037/dev0000292

Salanova, M., Llorens, S., & Cifre, E. (2013). The dark side of technologies: technostress among users of information and communication technologies. *Int. J. Psych. 48*(3). doi:10.1080/00207594.2012.680460

Sollisch, J. (2016, June 30). The cure for decision fatigue, *Wall Street Journal.* Retrieved from https://www.wsj.com/articles/the-cure-for-decision-fatigue-1465596928

Strayer, D. L., Drews, F.A., & Johnston, W. A. (2003). Cell phone-induced failures of visual attention during simulated driving. *Journal of Experimental Psychology: Applied, 9*(1) (pp. 23–32). https://doi.org/10.1037/1076-898X.9.1.23

Stroop, J. R. (1935). Studies of interference in serial verbal reactions. *Journal of Experimental Psychology, 18*(6) (pp. 643–662). doi:10.1037/h0054651. hdl:11858/00-001M-0000-002C-5ADB-7. Retrieved 2008-10-08.

Sweeten, G., Sillence, E., & Neave, N. (2018). Digital hoarding behaviours: Underlying motivations and potential negative consequences. *Computers in Human Behavior, 85* (pp. 54-60). doi:10.1016/j.chb.2018.03.031

Twenge, J. M. (2017). iGen: Why Today's Super-Connected Kids Are Growing Up Less Rebellious, More Tolerant, Less Happy and Completely Unprepared for Adulthood. ISBN: 978-1-5011-5201-6 paperback. (pp. 342). New York, NY

Twenge, J. M. (2017, September). Have Smartphones Destroyed a Generation? *The Atlantic,* https://www.theatlantic.com/magazine/archive/2017/09/has-the-smartphone-destroyed-a-generation/534198/

Twenge, J. M., Spitzberg, B. H., & Campbell, W. K. (2019, June). Less in-person social interaction with peers among U.S. adolescents in the 21st century and links to loneliness. *Journal of Social and Personal Relationships, 36*(6) (pp. 1892-1913). https://doi.org/10.1177/0265407519836170

van Bennekom, M. J., Blom, R. M., Vulink, N., & Denys, D. (2015). A case of digital hoarding.

Case Reports, http://dx.doi.org/10.1136/bcr-2015-210814.

Vohs, K. D., Baumeister, R. F., Schmeichel, B. J., Twenge, J. M., Nelson, N. M., & Tice, D. M. (2008, May). Making choices impairs subsequent self-control: a limited-resource account of decision making, self-regulation, and active initiative. *J Pers Soc Psychol, 94*(5) (pp. 883-98). doi: 10.1037/0022-3514.94.5.883. PMID: 18444745.

Vollrath, M., Schleicher, S., & Gelau, C. (2011). The influence of cruise control and adaptive cruise control on driving behaviour—A driving simulator study. *Accident Analysis & Prevention, 43*(3), (pp. 1134–1139). https://doi.org/10.1016/j.aap.2010.12.023

Wojcik, E. (Jan 2012). Students leave their iPods at home during 'crunch time'. *American Psychological Association (APA)* https://doi.org/10.1037/e740272011-003

Woollaston, V., (2013). How often do you check your phone? The average person does it 110 times a DAY (and up to every 6 seconds in the evening). *DailyMail.com.* Retrieved from https://www.dailymail.co.uk/sciencetech/article-2449632/How-check-phone-The-average-person-does-110-times-DAY-6-seconds-evening.html.

www.ingramcontent.com/pod-product-compliance
Lightning Source LLC
Chambersburg PA
CBHW071519220526
45472CB00003B/1077